CARDIAC DEFIBRILLATION – PREDICTION, PREVENTION AND MANAGEMENT OF CARDIOVASCULAR ARRHYTHMIC EVENTS

Edited by **Joyelle J. Harris**

Cardiac Defibrillation – Prediction, Prevention and Management of Cardiovascular Arrhythmic Events
Edited by Joyelle J. Harris

Published by InTech

Janeza Trdine 9, 51000 Rijeka, Croatia

Publishing Process Manager Romina Krebel

Technical Editor Teodora Smiljanic

Cover Designer InTech Design Team

Additional hard copies can be obtained from orders@intechopen.com

Cardiac Defibrillation – Prediction, Prevention and Management of Cardiovascular Arrhythmic Events, Edited by Joyelle J. Harris
p. cm.
ISBN 978-953-307-692-8

For EU product safety concerns:
IN TECH d.o.o., Prolaz Marije Krucifikse Kozulić 3, 51000 Rijeka, Croatia,
info@intechopen.com or visit our website at intechopen.com.

Meet the editor

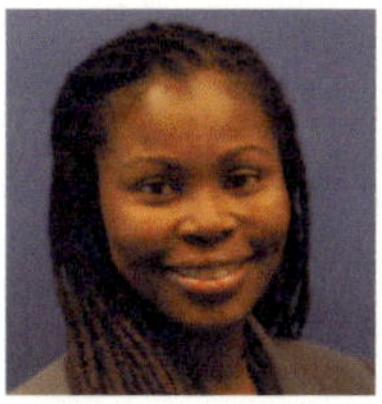

Dr. Harris earned her Ph.D. in electrical engineering from Princeton University in 2010. She specializes in stretchable electronic systems with medical device applications, and she has broad expertise in patterning electronic devices on unconventional substrates. Dr. Harris is currently a technical consultant in the Electrical and Semiconductor Practice at Exponent Engineering and Scientific Consulting firm. At Exponent she has partnered with the Biomechanics Practice to review and analyze pacemakers and implantable cardioverter defibrillators (ICDs). She is also a member of the battery task force where she analyzes cells for functionality and safety, and she conducts failure modes and effects analysis (FMEA). Dr. Harris has also examined methods of building water purification devices for residents of developing countries. Prior to joining Exponent, Dr. Harris worked as an electrical engineer at the American Competitiveness Institute in Philadelphia, PA. Dr. Harris has also worked at the Oak Ridge National Lab and the National Aeronautics and Space Administration (NASA).

Contents

Preface

Throughout the world, approximately 23 million people suffer from heart failure each year. Of all patients who experience heart failure, the mortality rate due to sudden cardiac death (SCD) is between 28% and 68%. SCD is most often due to ventricular tachycardia (VT) or ventricular fibrillation (VF). To alleviate SCD by VT and VF, one effective and common treatment is the use of implanted cardioverter-defibrillators (ICDs).

An ICD is a device that monitors the electrical activity of the user's heart and delivers an electrical shock upon detecting certain arrhythmias. While ICDs have decreased the number of deaths due to sudden cardiac arrhythmic events, studies suggests that patients with ICDs who receive shocks have a worse prognosis than similar patients who do not receive shocks.

These poor projections for patients who receive shocks are spurred by several factors. While the electrical shocks from ICDs save lives, they are also reported to be quite painful. Therefore, patients who have experienced a shock tend to suffer from psychological stress and a lower quality of life afterwards. Furthermore, about one third of ICD patients will experience inappropriate or unnecessary shocks from their ICDs. Inappropriate shocks have been linked to higher mortality rates in ICD patients. Other research suggests that after patients receive a shock, heart failure tends to progress more rapidly. Each of these factors highlights a gap in the body of knowledge relevant to ICDs. Therefore, a significant amount of research and clinical studies are needed to guarantee continued improvement for these devices.

One topic worthy of further exploration is the manner in which ICDs detect arrhythmias. At present, many ICDs use timing to classify heart rhythms. As a result, some safe rhythms are indistinguishable from life-threatening rhythms that have the same timing. For example, sinus tachycardia (ST) arrhythmia is safe and occurs during exercises in which the heart rate rises to about 120 beats per minute. On the other hand, ventricular tachycardia (VT) arrhythmia is fatal and occurs at the same heart rate. In spite of similar timing, ST and VT have different morphologies, suggesting that additional detection mechanisms could help avoid unnecessary shocks in ICD patients.

Another question to consider is how defibrillators can be employed to protect low risk patients from SCD. Patients who have a high risk of suffering from SCD are most likely identified by healthcare professionals, and then they receive life-saving ICDs. As a result, the majority of SCD victims are now low-risk patients because they remain unidentified and thus unprotected. A suggested answer to this quandary is to increase public access to defibrillators and to improve real-time, automated training on how to use such devices.

More research could also be done to determine ways of preventing shocks in ICD patients. For instance, examining the connection between diet, lifestyle, and ventricular arrhythmias could lead to such prevention. Diets rich in fish oils have shown promise in decreasing the risk of arrhythmatic cardiovascular events. However, to date, only a few studies have examined the use of fish oils to prevent ICD discharge. More studies could be done to increase this body of knowledge.

The chapters in this book explore the issues posed above in addition to discussing methods for improving ICDs and answering critical questions about ICD technology. The authors examine determinants for successful defibrillation and assess patients who receive defibrillation. Special cases in ICD patients are also considered along with clinical trials involving patients with defibrillators. The chapters presented herein contain a comprehensive overview of prediction, prevention, and management of cardiovascular events.

Joyelle J. Harris, Ph.D.
Exponent Failure Analysis Associates
Phoenix, Arizona
USA

Part 1

Defibrillation Introduction and Assessments

1

Implantable Cardioverter Defibrillators

Behzad Ghanavati
Department of Electrical Engineering, Mahshahr Branch, Islamic Azad University, Iran

1. Introduction

In recently years, Artificial Neural Networks have been studied extensively and applied in medical field, and have been demonstrated to have much better pattern recognition ability. In this chapter we present a VLSI chip to be implemented using 0.35 μm CMOS technology which is the implantable cardioverter defibrillator (ICDs).

Implantable cardioverter defibrillator is a device which monitors the heart and delivers electrical shock therapy in the event of a life-threatening arrhythmia.

At present most ICDs are often using time information from leads to classify rhythms. (Leong, P. H.W &Jabri, M.A November 1995) This means they cannot distinguish some dangerous rhythms from the safe one, as in the case of ventricular-tachycardia arrhythmia. (R. Coggins et al., 1995)

Our chip is used to distinguish between two types of arrhythmia; The Sinus Tachycardia (ST) arrhythmia and the Ventricular Tachycardia (VT) arrhythmia. The ST is a safe arrhythmia occurs during vigorous exercises and is characterized with rate of 120beat/minute. The VT is a fatal arrhythmia with the same rate. They can be separated only by detecting the morphology changes in each one. (Acherya,U,R.,2004)

Most morphology changes are appeared in the QRS-complex. The QRS-complex for both the ST and VT arrhythmia's are shown in fig.1. (Dale Dublin, 2000)

Since most morphology changes are appeared in the QRS-complex, for classifying the arrhythmias we must separate QRS complexes from ECG, consequently a new circuit for detecting QRS is designed. In this circuit the R-R distance between two QRS complexes and also the pulse width of QRS complex are used to improve the detection algorithm.

By using fuzzy logic and some parameters of ECG (pulse width, R-R interval and peak) we can separate QRS complex from ECG and after that apply this part to a Neural Network for classification.

The proposed analog VLSI chip can detect such morphology changes. It has the following advantages:

- It is easily interfaced to the analog signals in an ICD (in contrast to the digital systems which require analog to digital conversion).
- Analog circuits are generally small in area.
- Low voltage circuits are used to decrease battery weight and size and to extend battery life time which required for portable and modern wireless equipment.
- Hamming network did not need to have a training system and the reference vectors determine the weights.

- Although temperature variation is a major source of drift problems, no need for temperature compensation as the human body is considered a stable environment.

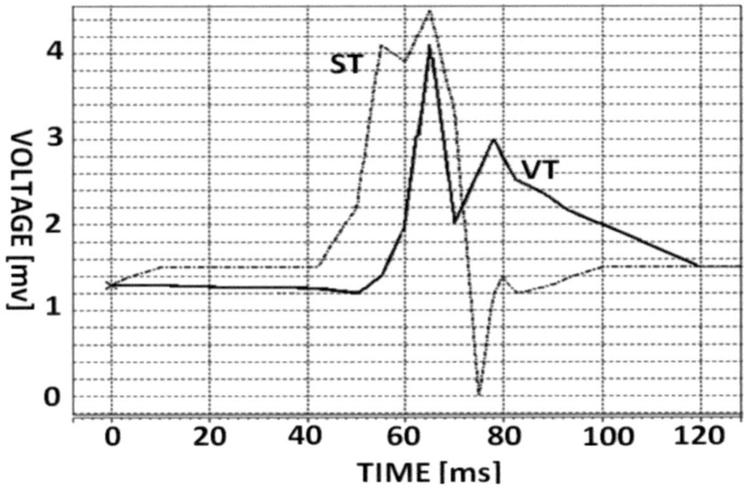

Fig. 1. Morphology change of QRS complex for both ST & VT.

This chapter deals with the design of Analog VLSI chip for implantable cardioverter defibrillator (ICDs). We first present the structure of system. Next, we describe each part separately and characteristic of each parts are described. Then, We show the circuits that are used for implementing of each part. Finally, we present the total block diagram of system with some simulations that verifies the functionality of system.

2. Architecture

The proposed chip consists of 3 main parts:

- QRS detector circuit
- Extracting QRS from an ECG circuit
- Classifying QRS complex circuit

First these parts will be explained separately and then the block diagram of the chip will be presented.

2.1 QRS detector circuit

The dominant component of the ECG is the QRS complex, which indicates the electrical depolarization of the muscles in the ventricle of the heart. Several clinical applications including implantable defibrillator require accurate QRS detection algorithms whiles The QRS is easily recognized by a human observer.

Various types of automated algorithms were proposed in the literature for detecting QRS. (K.Akazawa and K.Motoda 2001; Pan.J & Tompkins W.J 1985; Y. Suzuki, 1995) These algorithms use multiple features of the EGG including RR internal, pulse duration and amplitude, to detect QRS complexes. By processing several features, it is less likely that large amplitude but short duration noise would be mistaken for a QRS. Similarly, it is more likely that a true QRS with low amplitude, but normal width and RR internal would be correctly detected.

Fuzzy inference systems are well-suited for this application (fig.2), since detection in this system based on a few amounts of uncertainly which is very similar to the medical reasoning process.(O.Wieben, W.J Tompkins & V.X. Afonso 1999) Moreover the decision process is extremely easy to understand by human; consequently such easy interpretability allows external changes by experts on the decision process.

In this work, we are using a fuzzy inference system to identify QRS complexes. In this system QRS complex will be detected provided that a square wave synchronizes with them, consequently we use a fuzzy controller to adjust this square wave with QRS complexes.R-R internal, pulse duration and amplitude are features that enter to a controller as inputs parameter. Fuzzy controller evaluates these features and adjusts the output pulse of VCO to be synchronized with QRS complexes.

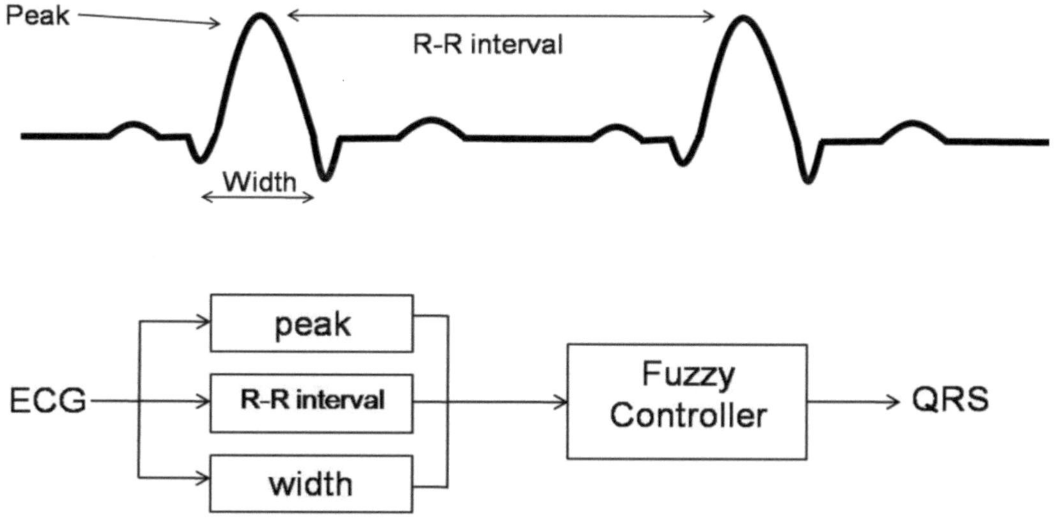

Fig. 2. QRS detection algorithm.

A feedback is used to correct the synchronization process. This feedback is produced by error between the output pulse of VCO and the pulse that show the width of QRS complex. This feedback is also enter to controller and processed by fuzzy controller. Finally, the output of fuzzy controller goes to VCO circuit and makes the output pulse of VCO to be synchronized with QRS complex (fig.3).

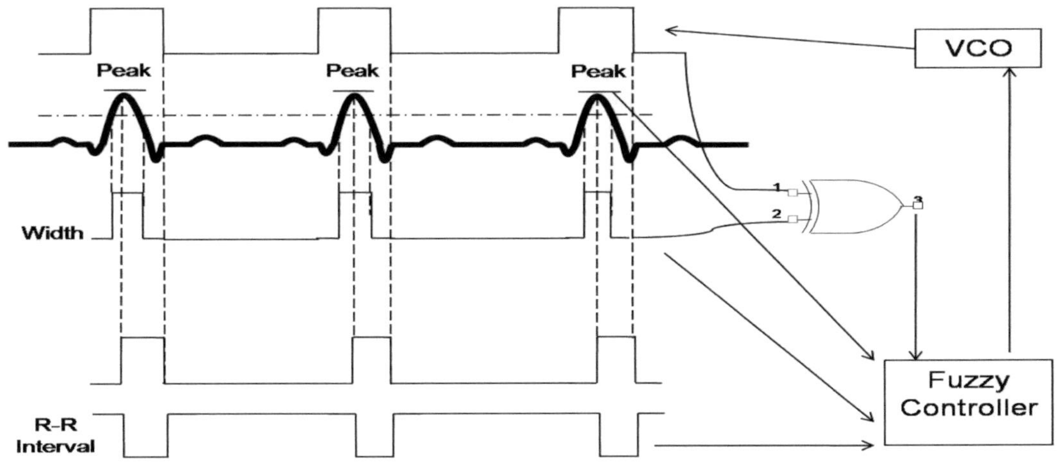

Fig. 3. QRS detection algorithms that is used in this project.

3. Extracting QRS from an ECG circuit

To separate QRS complexes, we passed ECG signals and synchronize VCO trough an analog median filter. (fig.4). Median Filter passes the median part of the input signals which, in this case, is QRS complexes.

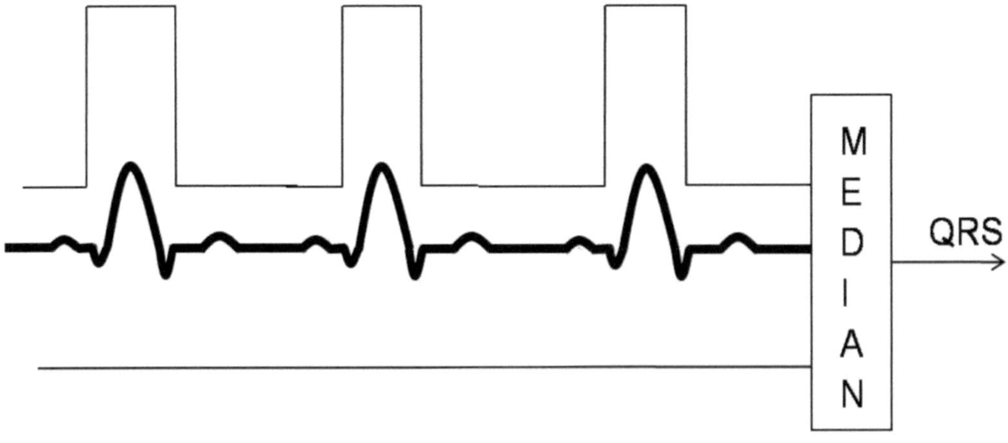

Fig. 4. Median Filter.

4. Classifying QRS complexes

The QRS complexes which were detected and separated from the rest of ECG signals are applied to an arrhythmia classifier. This classifier is used to distinguish between two types of arrhythmia: The Sinus Tachycardia (ST) arrhythmia and the Ventricular Tachycardia (VT) arrhythmia. The ST is a safe arrhythmia occurs during vigorous exercises and is characterized with rate of 120beat/minute. The VT is a fatal arrhythmia with the same rate. They can be separated only by detecting the morphology changes in each one.
Since the most morphology changes are appeared in the QRS complex, we apply QRS complex to an arrhythmia classifier to classify it. This arrhythmia classifier consists of three building blocks: a sample and hold (S/H) circuit, a mapping circuit and a Hamming neural network classifier. Fig.5 represents a block diagram of the chip. First, the rhythm is inputted to a sample and hold circuit to obtain 10 samples of the input signal. These 10 samples are inputted to mapping circuits in parallel to map into unit length [-1 1]. The outputs of mapping circuits are input to Hamming Neural Network, which has two neurons in its output layer. Each neuron responds to a specified type of the input arrhythmia.

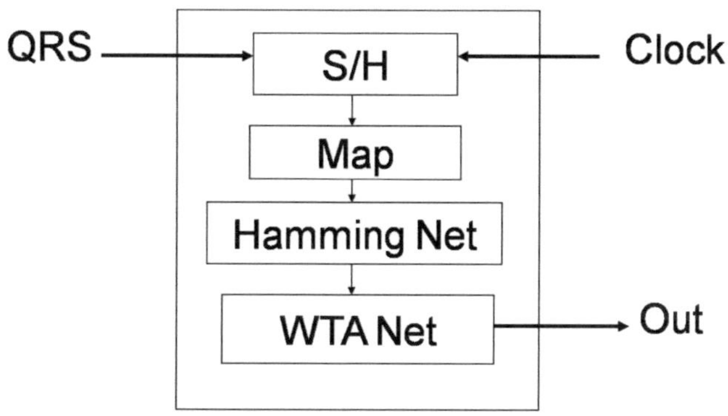

Fig. 5. Block diagram of QRS classifier.

4.1 Hamming Neural Network

A Neural Network classifier is made of a Hamming network, which is a maximum likelihood classifier network that can be used to determine which of several exemplar vectors are the most similar to an input vector (Laurene Fausett,1994 & M. B. Menhaj,2000). Fig.6 shows the simplest structure of a competitive layer.

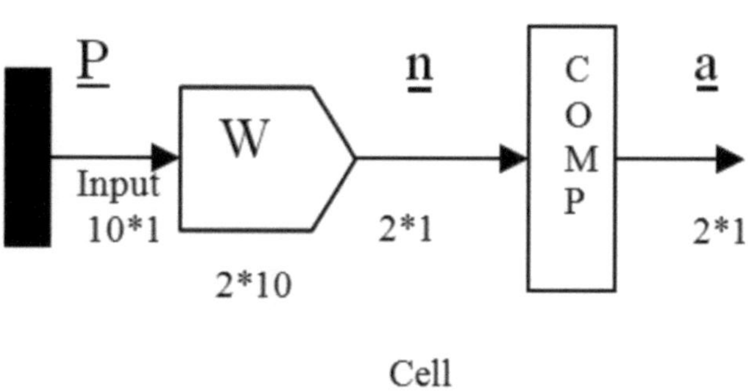

Fig. 6. A competitive cell.

$$\underline{a} = comp(W\underline{P}) \tag{1}$$

$$a_i = \begin{cases} 1, & i = i^* \\ 0, & i \neq i^* \end{cases} \tag{2}$$

i* is number of the cell that has the highest n_i for our application i=1, 2.
In the Hamming Network, reference vector determines the weights (w) of the network.The hamming distance between input vector ($\underline{P}$) and reference vector is calculated by $\underline{n}$ vector (equation 3). (Laurene Fausett,1994 & M. B. Menhaj, 2000)
Winner cell is determined with multiplying input vector to weights. The largest value corresponds to the smallest angle between input and weights vector if they are both of unit length [-1 1] (Laurene Fausett,1994 & M. B. Menhaj, 2000).

$$\underline{n} = W\underline{P} = \begin{bmatrix} W_{11} & W_{12} & .... & W_{110} \\ W_{21} & W_{22} & .... & W_{210} \end{bmatrix} \underline{P} = \begin{bmatrix} \cos\ \theta_1 \\ \cos\ \theta_2 \end{bmatrix} \tag{3}$$

5. Circuit design

The designing method of blocks show in fig.5 is given below:

5.1 Sample and hold (S&H) circuit

The Sample and hold delay circuit is made of 10 cascaded stages to obtain 10 samples of the input pulse. Fig. 7 shows S/H circuit.

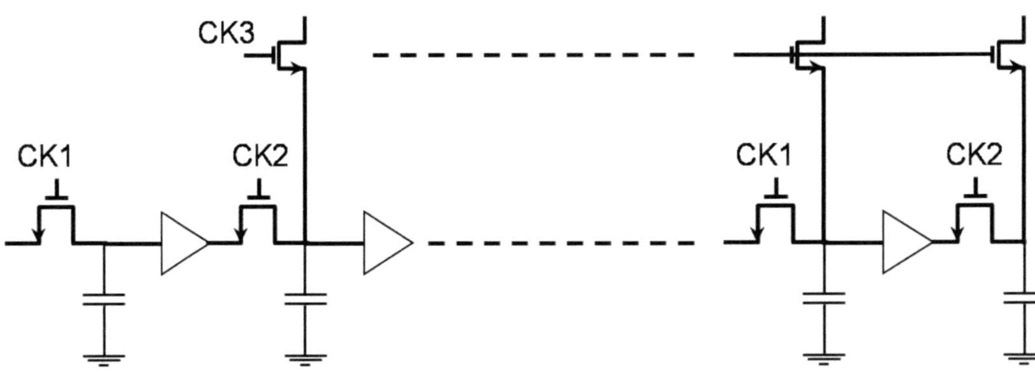

Fig. 7. Three stages of S/H circuit.

Two-phase non-overlapping clock (CK_1,CK_2) is used to control S/H. The sampled signal x_i then are inputted mapping circuit through another analog switch m_i controlled by CK_3. The timing diagram of CK_1, CK_2, CK_3 and the simulation result of the 1st stage of sample and hold circuit are shown in fig. 8.

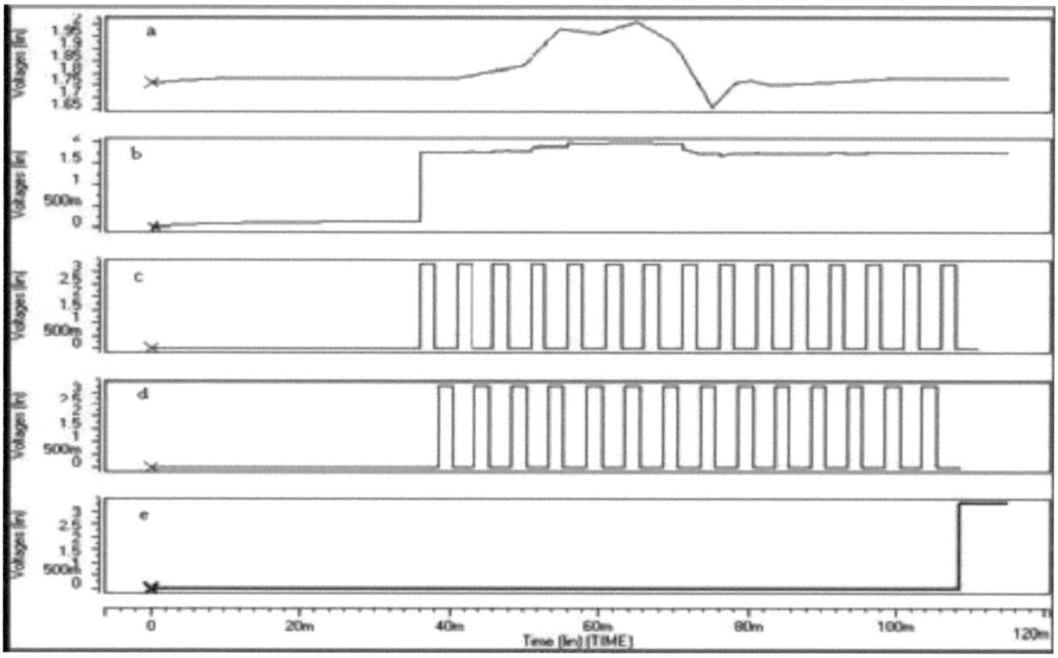

Fig. 8. (a) Input to S/H circuit. (b) Sampling signal of the 1st stage. (c) CK1. (d) CK2. (e) CK3.

In Fig. 8, the input rhythm of ST is applied to the S/H circuit and output of 1st stage is shown.

5.2 Mapping circuit

Before applying sampled data to Neural Network We have to map them into unit length [-1 1]. Figure 9 shows schematic of mapping circuit.

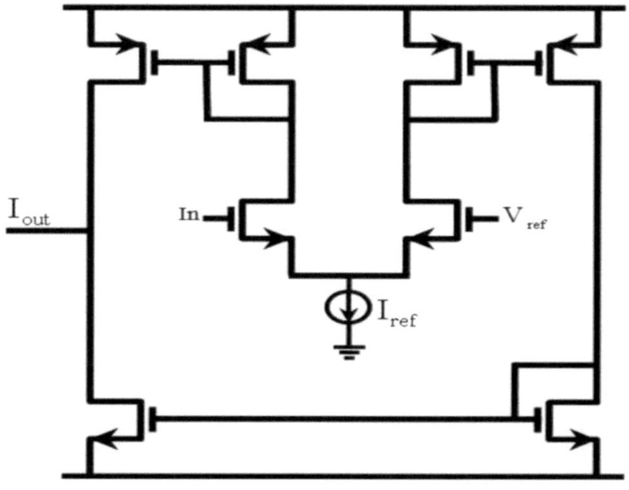

Fig. 9. Mapping circuit.

We use a simple differential pair in order to map input signal (sampled data) to unit length space [-1, 1]. By changing V_{ref} and W/L ratio of input stage of differential pair, we can map any space to unit length space. (Wilamowski, B 1999)

5.3 Hamming Neural Network classifier

The Hamming Network consists of two groups of synapses and two layers of neurons. The first group with weight vector W_1= (W_{11}, W_{12}, W_{13}, …, W_{115}) is connected to first neuron layer. The second layer with weight vector W_2= (W_{21}, W_{22}, W_{23}, …, W_{215}) is connected to second neuron layer, each neuron in the output layer responds to a specified class of input arrhythmia. Figure 10 shows the structure of Network

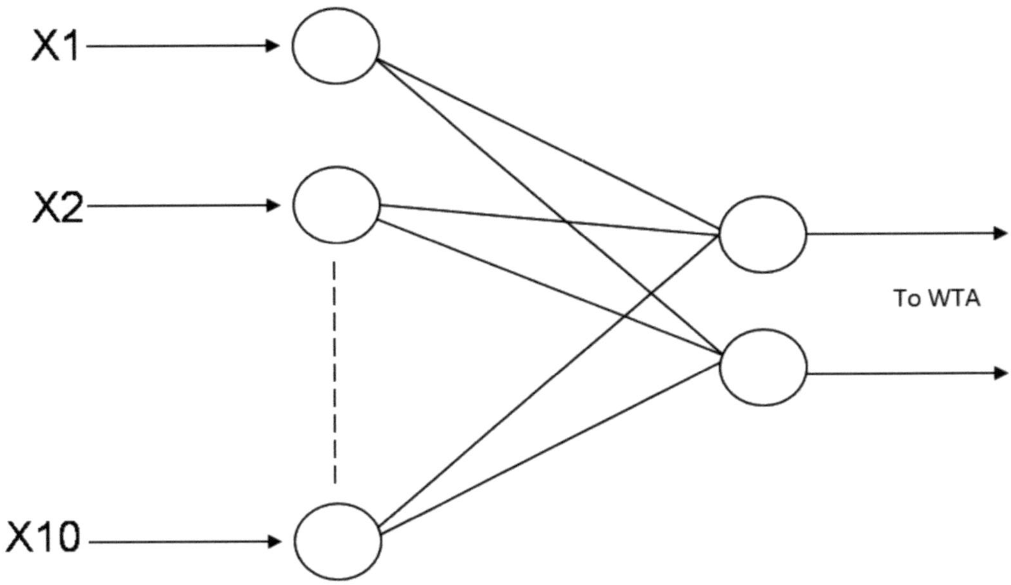

Fig. 10. Hamming Neural Network.

5.3.1 Synapse

The computation of inner product between input signal and the local interconnection weight is called synapse and is mostly done by using an analog multiplier.(S. T.Lee; H. Shawkey 1999)

We use a new low voltage low power four quadrant analog multiplier as a synapse. Since output of a synapse is current, output of 10 synapses can be summed at a single node of circuit.

The circuit consists of four quadratic cells is shown in figure 11 where the relationship between the input current, I_{in}, and the output current, I_{out}, are quadratic. The quadratic cell is made of two transistors M_n and M_p which are biased to operate in triode region and M_c which operates at saturation region.

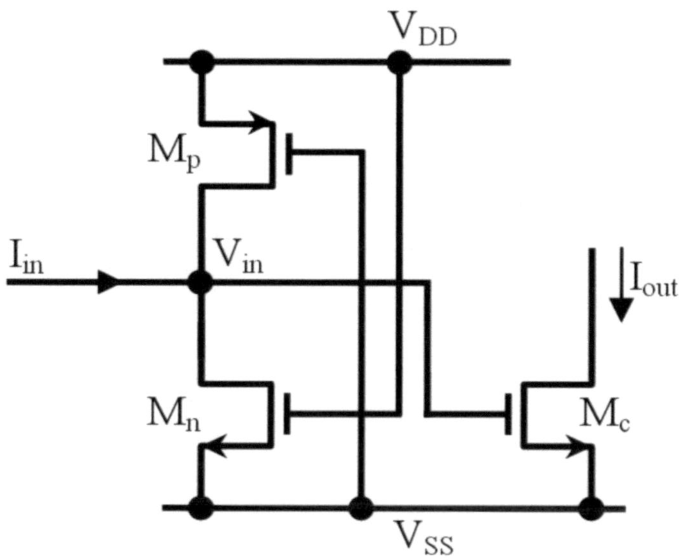

Fig. 11. Quadratic cell.

If M_n and M_p have the same transconductance, $\left(k_p = \mu_p C_{ox}\frac{W}{L} = k_n = \mu_n C_{ox}\frac{W}{L} = k\right)$ Then, it can be easily shown that the voltage (V_{in}) and the current (I_{out}) are given by

$$V_{in} = aI_{in} + b \tag{4}$$

$$I_{out} = k\left(c + I_{in}\right)^2 \tag{5}$$

Where a, b and c are $\dfrac{1}{k(2V_{DD} - |V_{tp}| - V_{tn})}, \dfrac{V_{DD}(V_{tn} - |V_{tp}|)}{2V_{DD} - |V_{tp}| - V_{tn}}$ and $\dfrac{2V_{DD}(V_{DD} - |V_{tp}|)}{2V_{DD} - |V_{tp}| - V_{tn}} - V_{tn}$ respectively.

Figure 12 shows the proposed four quadrant current multiplier circuit. The input currents of a multiplier are the sum of currents I_X and I_Y and the subtraction of the input currents I_X and I_Y. By using quadratic relationship between input and output currents which are derived from Equation (5) drain currents of M_{C1}, M_{C2}, M_{C3} and M_{C4} would be

$$I_{C1} = k[c + a(I_X + I_Y)]^2 \tag{6}$$

$$I_{C2} = k[c - a(I_X + I_Y)]^2 \tag{7}$$

$$I_{C3} = k[c + a(I_X - I_Y)]^2 \tag{8}$$

$$I_{C4} = k[c - a(I_X - I_Y)]^2 \tag{9}$$

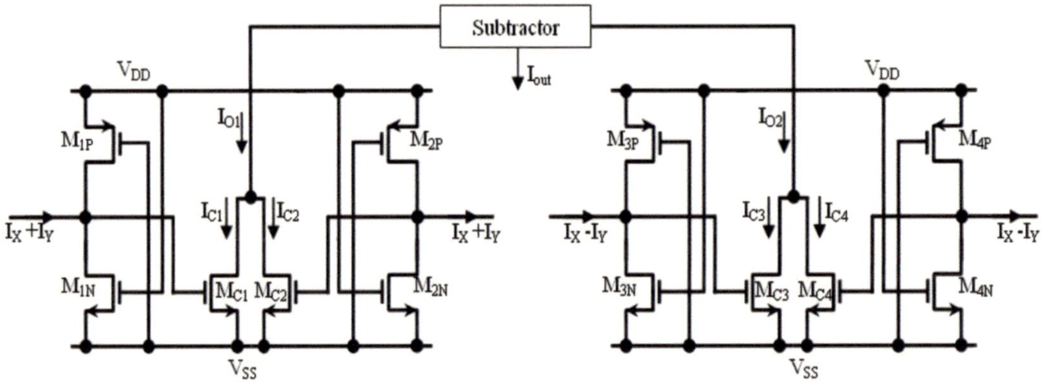

Fig. 12. Multiplier as a synapse.

According to Fig. 12, I_{O1} is the combination of I_{C1} and I_{C2} while I_{O2} is the combination of I_{C3} and I_{C4}. I_{O1} and I_{O2} can be shown as

$$I_{O1} = k[2c^2 + 2a^2(I_X + I_Y)^2] \tag{10}$$

$$I_{O2} = k[2c^2 + 2a^2(I_X - I_Y)^2] \tag{11}$$

The output current of the four quadrant current multiplier I_{out} is the difference between I_{O1} and I_{O2} and is given by

$$I_{OUT} = I_{O1} - I_{O2} = 8ka^2 I_X I_Y \tag{12}$$

Fig. 13 Shows DC characteristic of current multiplier circuit under input current ranging from -20 µA to 20 µA.

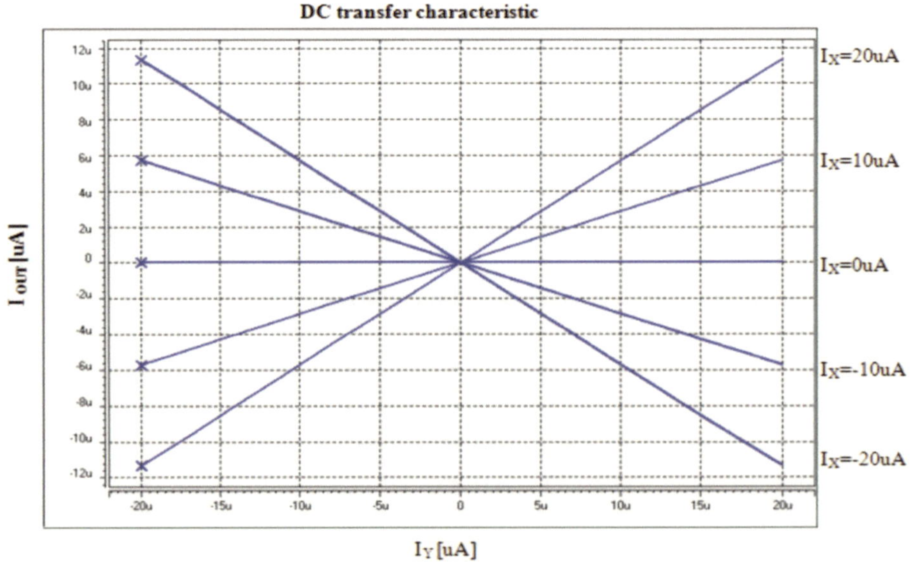

Fig. 13. DC transfer characteristic of four quadrant current multiplier.

5.3.2 Winner take all

The function of the WTA is to accept input signals, compare their values and produce a high digital output value (logic 'one') corresponding to the largest input, while all other digital outputs are set to low output value (logic 'zero').(J.Ramirez-Angulo et al., 2005)
Fig. 14 shows the block diagram of the WTA circuit. The circuit includes a 2-input current maximum selector with a simple voltage inverter.(.Ramirez-Angulo et al., 2005)

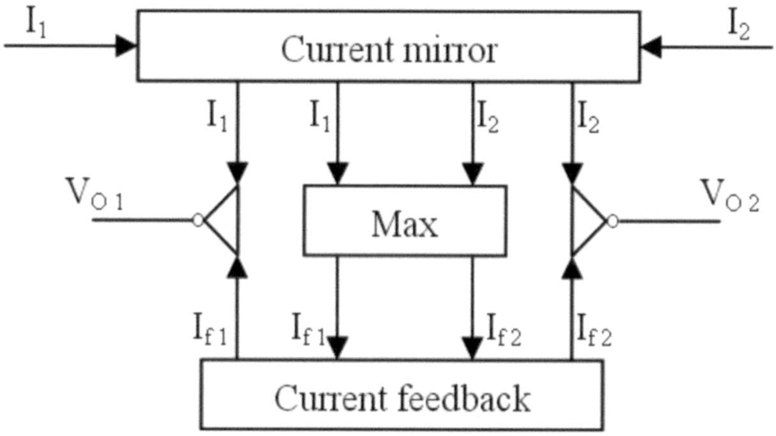

Fig. 14. Winner take all circuit.

5.3.3 The current max selector

The 2-input current maximum selector is shown in Fig. 15. The proposed current max selector has 2 input branches and each branch consists of an FVF (R.G. Carvajal et al., 2005), which is formed by voltage follower M_{ai}, and current sensing transistor M_{ci}.

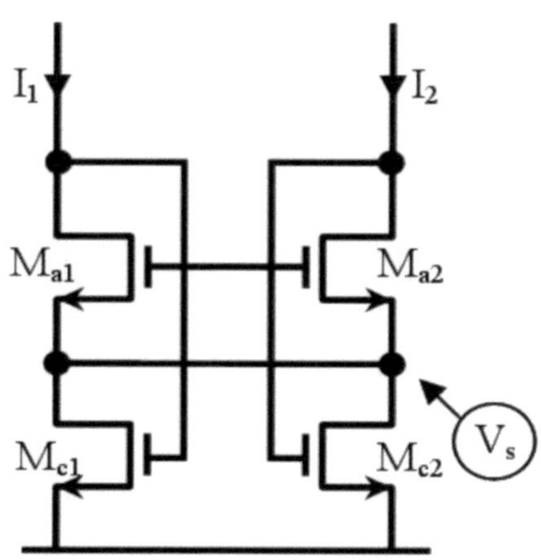

Fig. 15. 2-input max circuit.

Transistor M_{ai} in an FVF performs as an improved voltage follower and the Gate-Source voltage drop of this transistor is constant (neglecting second-order effect) and independent of the load.
Transistor M_{ci} operates as a current sensing device. It can sink large current by keeping its Drain voltage approximately constant. Moreover, the existing impedance at the Source of transistor M_{ai} is very low due to the feedback loop.
The principle of operation of the circuit is as follow. The voltage at node "V_S" follows the maximum of input currents I_1, I_2, with a DC level shift V_{GSn} where n denotes the maximum current.
In this condition the transistor (M_{a1} or M_{a2}) which carrying the minimum current, has the greater Gate-Source voltage than the value that should have to operate in saturation mode, at this condition this transistor operates in triode mode with Drain-Source voltage value close to zero, thus the current sensing transistor is turning off in this branch and minimum and maximum currents passed through current sensing transistor of winning branch due to properties of FVF cell.

5.3.4 The overall structure of WTA circuit

The circuit of the 2-input WTA is shown in Fig.16. The currents (I_1, I2) are the inputs of the circuit.
Each current is mirrored into current max Selector, as well as, into the feedback circuit due to PMOS current mirror M_{12}, M_{22}.
Thus the input current of each voltage inverter is:

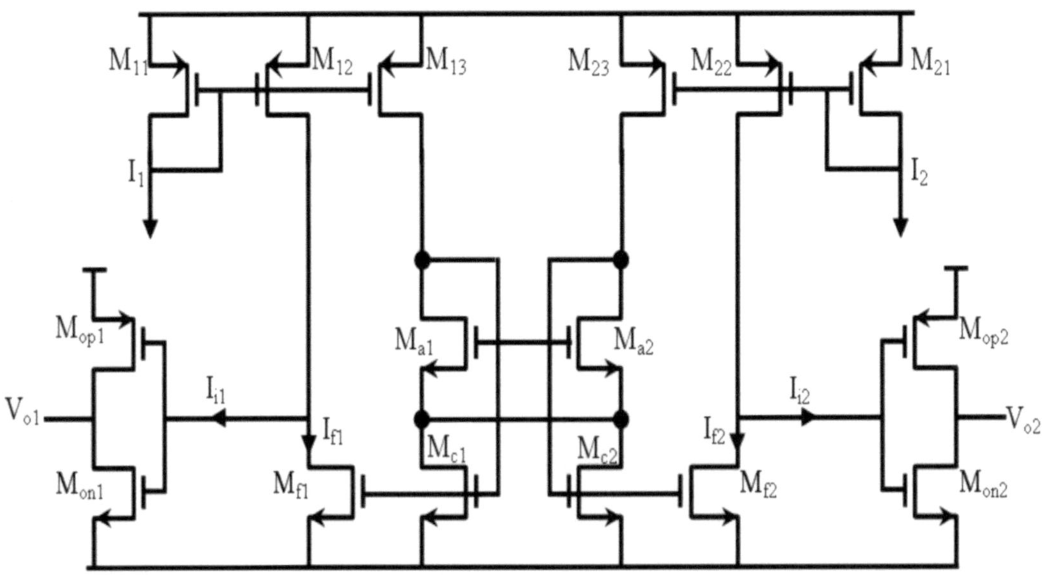

Fig. 16. 2-input WTA circuit.

$$I_{i1} = I_1 - I_{f1} \tag{13}$$

$$I_{i2} = I_2 - I_{f2} \tag{14}$$

We assume at the steady state, the current I_1 is the largest input current I_1=max (I_1, I_2)
So

$$I_{f1} = I_1 + I_2 \tag{15}$$

$$I_{f2} = 0 \tag{16}$$

From the Equation (13) - Equation (16) the input current of each voltage inverter is:

$$I_{i1} = I_1 - (I_1 + I_2) = -I_2 \tag{17}$$

$$I_{i2} = I_2 - 0 = I_2 \tag{18}$$

This means that only one input current of the voltage inverter, which is correspond to minimum current, is positive and all the other currents are negative. Thus the digital voltage outputs of the circuit will be at logic

$$\begin{cases} V_{o1} = \text{'one'} \\ V_{o2} = \text{'zero'} \end{cases} \tag{19}$$

Fig.17 shows the block diagram of the proposed QRS classifier

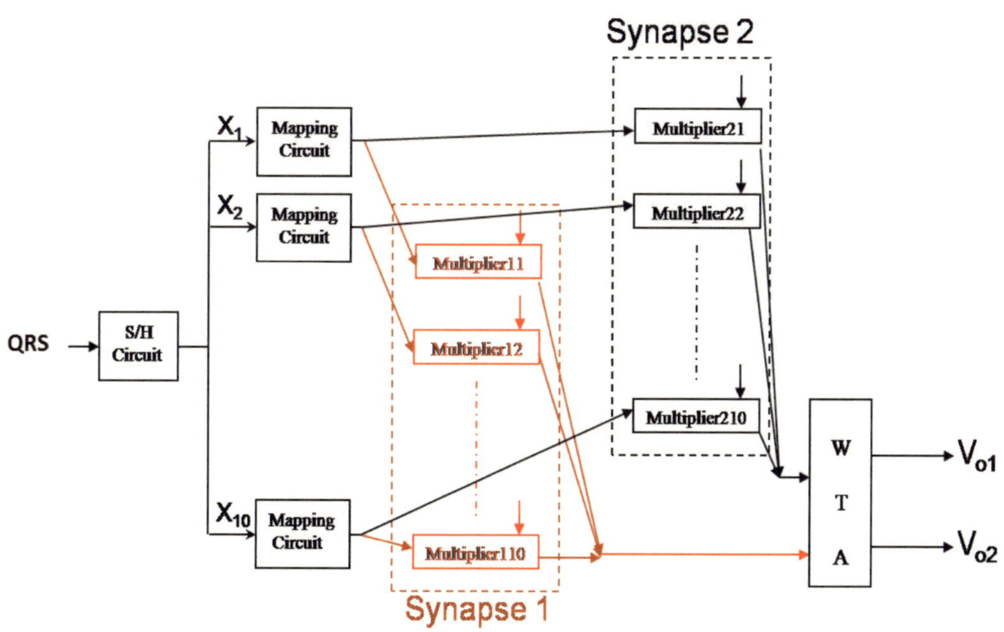

Fig. 17. Block diagram of the proposed QRS classifier.

6. The proposed arrhythmia classifier chip

The block diagram of proposed system is presented in fig.18.
In this system, multiple features of ECG are measured by analog circuit. These features are applied to a fuzzy controller to be processed. The output of fuzzy controller goes to a VCO which is used to synchronize the output pulse of VCO with the specific part of ECG. Finally, the QRS complexes which are filtered by median filter are applied to arrhythmia classifier provided that the error of detection algorithm is below a normal value. Moreover, the arrhythmia classifier has 2 outputs that each one responds to a specific type of the input arrhythmia.

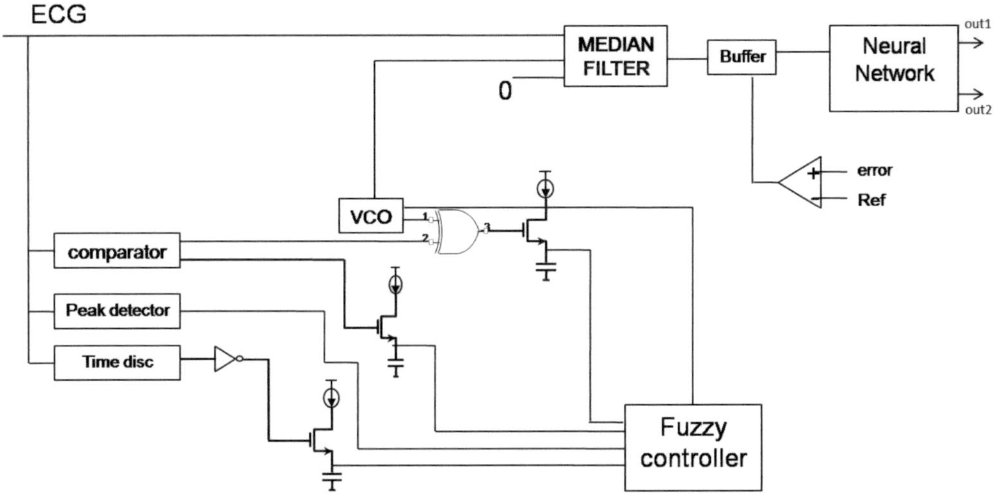

Fig. 18. Block diagram of proposed system.

Simulation result of the system in both cases is shown in figure 19 and 20.
In fig.19 the inputting rhythm of ST is applied to system caused to digital outputs of OUT1 goes to "One" and OUT2 goes to" Zero".

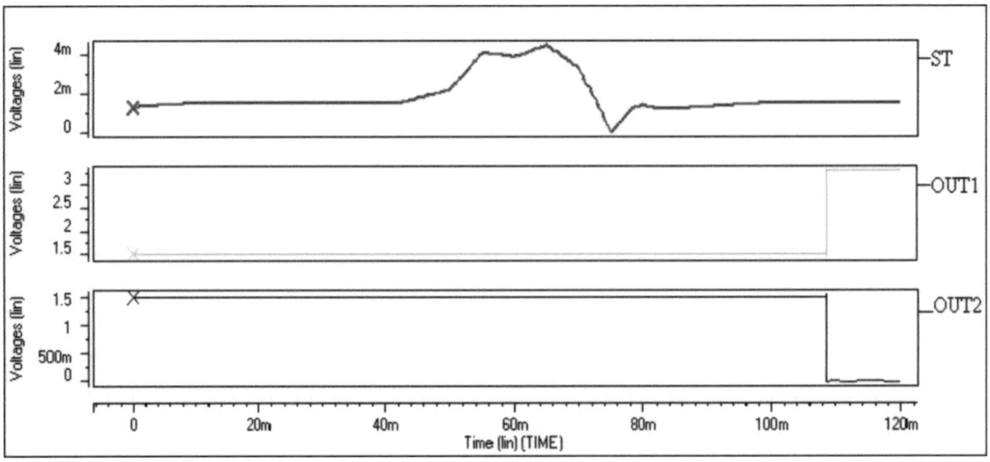

Fig. 19. Output of system for ST input.

In fig.20 the inputting rhythm of VT is applied to system caused to digital outputs of OUT1 goes to "Zero" and OUT2 goes to "One".

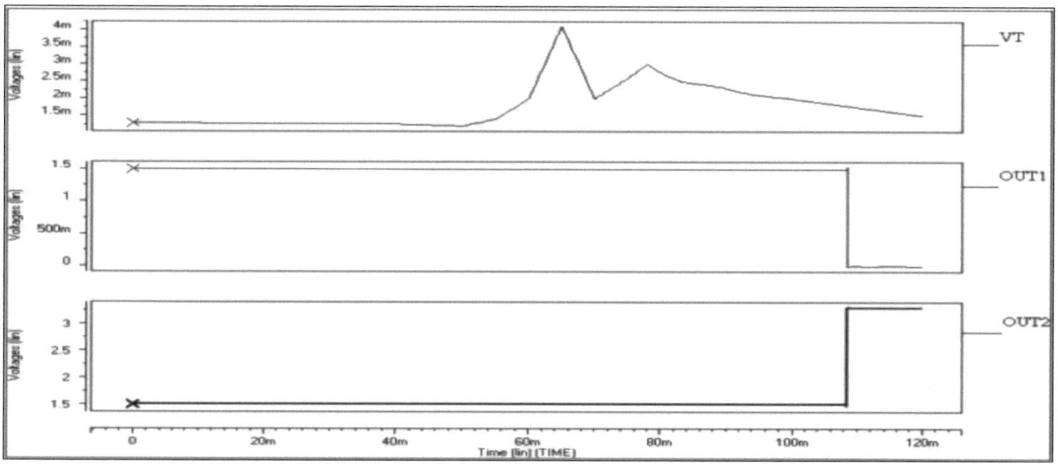

Fig. 20. Output of system for VT input.

7. Conclusion

In this chapter a VLSI Analog chip for arrhythmia classification is presented.
The proposed Network has the following features:

- No need for A/D converter between the ECG and the classification system.
- The system operates in the low frequency range, so that the parasitic of the layout likely have no effect on the operation of the chip.
- This system can be extended to distinguish m types of arrhythmias by using m number of neurons in the output layer of the Hamming Neural Network circuit.

8. References

Leong, P. H.W and Jabri, M.A (November 1995) *A low power VLSI Arrhythmia classifier* IEEE Transaction on Neural Networks volume 6, Page(s):1435-1445

R. Coggins, M. Jabri, B. Flower and S.'Pickard (June 1995.) *A low- Power Network for On-Line Diagnosis of Heart Patients*Trans. IEEE Micro, pp. 18-25

Acherya,U,R. (2004) *Classification of cardiac abnormalities using heart rate signal* Med and Bio Eng, vol 42, P.288-293

Dale Dublin (2000) *Rapid Interpretation of EKG* McGraw-Hill

O.Wieben, W.J Tompkins and V.X. Afonso (1999) *classification of PVCS with a fuzzy logic system* IEEE Trans. Biomed. Eng,vol 38, pp.561-570,

Y. Suzuki (November 1995) *Self organizing QRS-wave recognition in ECG using neural networks* IEEETrans. Neural network, Vo1.6, No.6, pp. 1469-1477,

Pan.J and Tompkins W.J (1985) *a real-time QRS detection algorithm* IEEE Trans. Biomed. Eng,vol BME 32, n3, pp.230-236

K.Akazawa and K.motoda (September 2001) *Adaptive threshold QRS detection algorithm for ambulatory ECG* IEEE computer in cardiology, pp.445-448,

H. Shawkey, H. Elsimary, H. Haddara, H.F. Ragaie,(1999) *Design of a VLSI Neural Network Arrhythmia Classifier* Proceeding of the sixteenth National Radio Science conference, NRSC'99. Egypt, page(s): C 27/1-C 2710

Laurene Fausett (1994) *fundamental of Neural Network*. Prentice Hall

M. B. Menhaj (2000) *Computational intelligence (vol1): Fundamental of Neural Networks,* Amirkabir center of Publishing,

Behzad Razavi (2000) *Design of Analog CMOS integrated circuits,* McGraw-Hill,

Du Chen, John G. Harris, Jose C.Principe (2004) *A Bio-amplifier with pulse output* Proceeding 26th Annual international conference of the Engineering in Medicine and Biology Society. EMBC volume2, page(s):4071-4074 vol.6

Wilamowski, B. M and Jaeger, R.C and Kaynak, M. O(December 1999) *Neuro-Fuzzy Architecture for CMOS Implementation* IEEE Trans Industrial Electronics. Volume 46. Issue 6.page(s):1132-1136

F. A. Salam and M. R. Choi(1991), *Analog MOS Vector multipliers for the implementation of synapses in artificial neural networks* Journal of Circuits, Systems, and Computers, vol. 1, no, 2, pp. 205-228.

S. T.Lee and K. T. Lau (1999) *A reconfigurable Low-voltage low-power building block for Artificial Neural Network* Proc. Int. Conf. on Neural Networks. Volume 3, page(s): 1478-1481, vol.3.

S. vlassis and S. siskos (1999) *High speed and high resolution WTA circuit* Proceedings of the 1999 IEEE international symposium on circuits and systems.ICAS'99.volume 2 page(s):224-227

J.Ramirez-Angulo, G.Ducodray-Acevedo, R. G. Carjaval, A. Lopez-Martin (June 2005) *Low-voltage high-performance voltage-mode and current-mode WTA circuit based on flipped voltage followers* IEEE Trans. Circuits Syst. II, Express Briefs, vol. 52,no. 7.

R.G. Carvajal, J. Ramírez-Angulo, A. López-Martin, A.Torralba, J. Galán, A. Carlosena and F. Muñoz1 (July 2005)*The Flipped Voltage Follower: A Useful Cell for Vow-Voltage Low-Power Circuit design* IEEE Transactions on Circuits and Systems I,Vol. 52, No.7

2

Defibrillation Shock Amplitude, Location and Timing

Shimon Rosenheck
Hadassah Hebrew University Medical Center, Jerusalem, Israel

1. Introduction

The only effective treatment of ventricular fibrillation, in both clinical and experimental medicine, is the electrical defibrillation. Although, critical site ablation is feasible in idiopathic ventricular fibrillation (Knecht et al, 2009), the defibrillation still has remained the only evidence based, generally accepted treatment of this arrhythmia (Jacobs et al, 2010; Deakin et al, 2010). Strong evidence supports that external and internal defibrillations can save the life of patient at risk for sudden cardiac death. Several high-risk groups were defined and implantable defibrillators significantly prolonged the life of these patients when compared to the best medical treatment (Maron, 2002; Ezekowitz et al, 2003; Desai et al, 2004; Dalal et al, 2005; Silka et al, 2006; Sacher et al, 2006; Daubert et al, 2007; Rosenheck et al, 2010). However, the majority of sudden cardiac death victims belong to the low-risk groups. For this reason, most of the sudden cardiac death cases cannot be protected with implantable defibrillators (Huikuri et al, 2001). To resolve this paradox, public access defibrillation was suggested in the high-risk locations (Folk et al, 2010; Winkle et al, 2010; Kitamura et al, 2010; Eisenberg et al, 2010; Rho et al, 2011). Moreover, most of the sudden cardiac death cases occur at home, mainly during the early morning hours. Only early defibrillation may save these patients and to achieve it defibrillators will be available in each house. Non-professional persons, who may witness the sudden cardiac death, will operate these home-defibrillators. They cannot verify the success of the intervention and cannot react immediately with a second shock if the fibrillation continues after the first one and the defibrillator will not detect the failure. For this reason, the successful defibrillation with the first shock is even more important and the external defibrillators will be necessarily more reliable and user-friendly (Rosenheck et al, 2009a).
During the last 25 years, a vast amount of information on clinical and experimental defibrillation was accumulated. The experimental data was obtained from the effect of shock on single cell, in small-perfused tissues and whole heart. Until recently, the available methods did not allow imaging of defibrillation in closed chest models. Mathematical simulations contributed to the understanding of ventricular fibrillation mechanism and defibrillation in closed chest models and human subjects.
External and internal factors determine the defibrillation success or failure. Usually, the external factors, like shock amplitude, location and timing may be modified. These factors belong to the physical properties of the defibrillators. A computerized automatic defibrillator has to be flexible, and capable to deliver the most effective defibrillation shock

when needed. These 3 properties may be integrated and personalized for each individual patient. However, the location and timing are still not used in the available defibrillators. The only controllable parameter, in both internal and external defibrillators, is the amplitude of the delivered shock and it may be unnecessarily very high. The possible combination of these external shock characteristics will be discussed.
It is more difficult to control the internal than the external factors. This is the reason for occasional non-reproducibility of the defibrillation outcome in the same subject with the same shock setting. The propagation of the ventricular fibrillation waveform prior to the defibrillation, the state of depolarization of the myocardium, spiral waves and singularity points or lines are only a few of many known and still unknown factors. These internal determinants will also be discussed and correlated to the above-mentioned external factors.

2. Shock amplitude – Historical and clinical data

More than 100 years ago, it was discovered that a shock might terminate ventricular arrhythmias. Already at that time it was understood that only a strong shock might be successful. Many theories were proposed to explain the mechanism of the defibrillation. All these theories offered reason for the need of a high energy for defibrillations. The first theory was proposed by Wiggers and was called the "Total Extinction" hypothesis (Wiggers, 1940). According to it, the energy delivered to the fibrillating heart has to be able to terminate the electrical activity of the whole myocardium, to create a silent period, and to allow the normal rhythm to overtake the electrical activity in the heart muscle. Wiggers sustained that maintaining the fibrillation even in a small mass of myocardium will prevent resumption of the coordinated activity. Although there is a strong logic in this hypothesis and is simple and attractive, future experimental evidences did not support it. First of all, there is no need to terminate the electrical activity in all the myocardial mass. It is enough to defibrillate only a certain amount of the fibrillating myocardium and the arrhythmia in the rest of the myocardium is not enough to continue the fibrillation. This hypothesis is called the "Critical Mass" hypothesis (Zipes et al, 1975). Moreover, it is not enough only to terminate the arrhythmia, but also it is important to avoid reinitiation of the fibrillation (Trayanova et al, 2006). Regardless the hypothesis, only a strong shock can terminate and prevent re-induction of ventricular fibrillation.

2.1 Defibrillation dose-response curve

Because the only measurable parameter was the amplitude of the shock, different methods were suggested to correlate the shock energy with the success of the defibrillation. This correlation between the defibrillation energy and the defibrillation success is a sigmoid dose-response curve (Figure 2.1). At a low energy a small percent of the attempts may still be successful and the success rate will increase with stronger shocks. The curve achieves a theoretical plateau at certain energy. As long as the defibrillation was achieved with an external defibrillator under professional human control, this dose response curve had only theoretical and academic importance. With the introduction of implantable automatic defibrillators, the energy had to be programmed from a head, considering the required success rate of >99%.
In an experimental study, to obtain a dose-response curve, 48 trials had to be performed, during 192 minutes (Davy et al, 1987). Although this method is the most reliable to determine the safe programmed energy, it is not acceptable for clinical evaluation. After

induction of ventricular fibrillation, either intra-operative or at a latter test of the defibrillation threshold, repeated tests each one with a lower shock-energy are performed. The testing is stopped when the defibrillation fails and the last successful defibrillation energy is considered the defibrillation threshold. In experimental models this energy will be able to defibrillate only 50%-75% of the episodes. The safe energy to program the first shock of the automatic defibrillator is the plateau energy and this is achieved by doubling the threshold energy. The desired clinical test is shown in Figure 2.2, but the practiced clinical protocols are shown in Figure 2.3. These tests were used during the last 20 years. Today, because the big gap between the threshold and the device capacity, the number of shocks used for the test is reduced to minimum and even it is seriously questioned (Higgins et al, 2005; Viskin & Rosso, 2008).

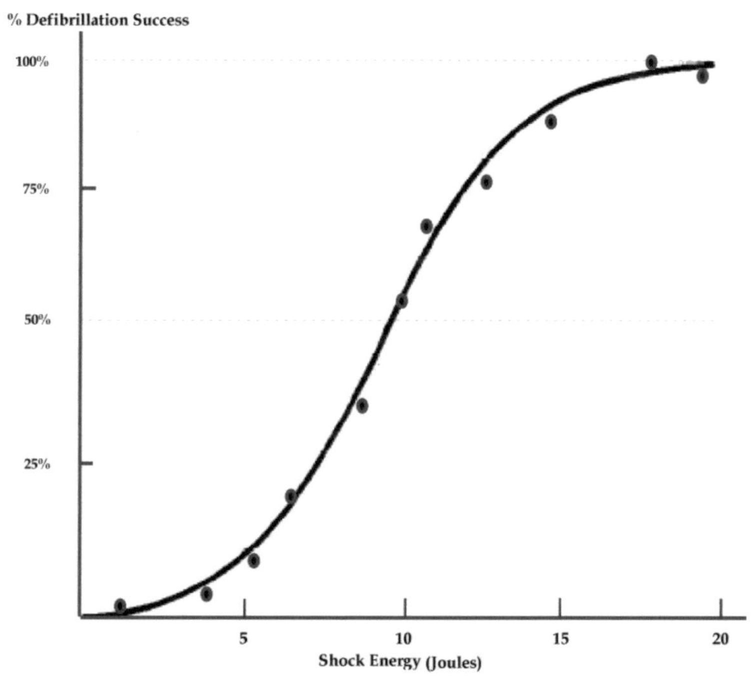

Fig. 2.1. The sigmoid-dose response curve showing nonlinear correlation between the defibrillation success and the delivered shock energy. This correlation is reproducible (see text). To achieve a higher defibrillation success the energy level has to be increased. There is a saturation level above which practically all the attempts will be successful. Per definition only 50% of the attempts will be defibrillated successfully at the threshold value. With a defibrillation energy twice higher than the threshold value the success rate is above 90%.

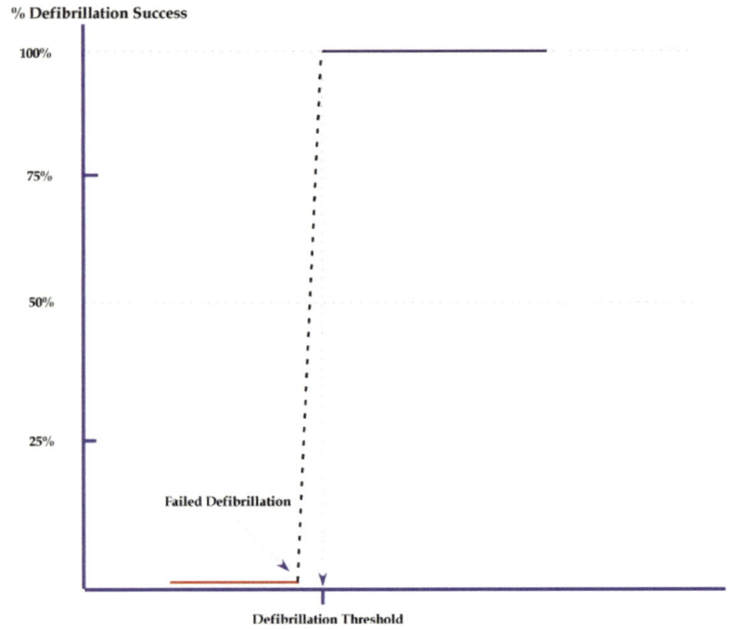

Fig. 2.2. The desired clinical defibrillation threshold testing. The immediately higher energy before the first failed attempt is considered the defibrillation threshold.

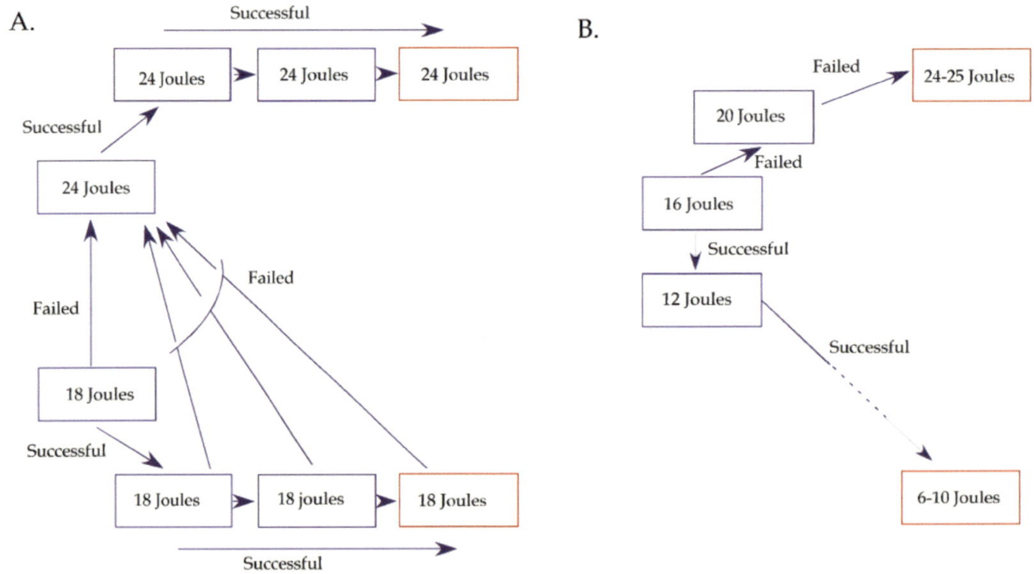

Fig. 2.3. Clinical protocols. A. Two-step fortified test. B. Multi-step test. For both test the last effective defibrillation energy is considered the DFT or best-predicted DFT (DFT-defibrillation threshold). If the highest acceptable energy is not effective, lead revision is recommended or addition of subcutaneous lead system. Today a single energy test is recommended (see text). Moreover, there is no unanimous agreement on the necessity of DFT testing at all (see text).

When the more simplified defibrillation threshold testing (Figure 2.3B) was compared with the dose-response curve, the ED_{50} (the energy with 50% defibrillation success rate) was similar with the defibrillation threshold described above (Jones, 1991). Subsequently, more limited test (Figure 2.3A) was suggested and extensively used in clinical practice. This testing is based on induction of ventricular fibrillation and defibrillation with the same shock energy at least 3-4 times, consecutively (Figure 2.3A). If during one of the tests the defibrillation failed, a higher energy was tested, again 3-4 times. If the first energy was successful at all the attempts, it was accepted as the defibrillation threshold. If a higher energy was successful in all the consecutive tests, this energy was accepted as the defibrillation threshold, but only if a 10 Joules margin between this value and the device's maximal capacity was maintained. If the defibrillation with the highest acceptable energy was not successful, lead revision was required. Although this method may not offer the same accuracy as the dose-response curve or the limited defibrillation threshold testing (Figure 2.3B), it was reliable, predictive and the long-term survival of these patients was not affected (Rosenheck et al, 2009b). After implementation of the biphasic shock (Bardy et al, 1989) and the unipolar defibrillation system (Bardy et al et al, 1993) in the implantable defibrillators, the defibrillation threshold decreased much below the device capacity and testing with single defibrillation attempt is justified (Higgins et al, 2005). Moreover, as previously mentioned, the need of testing was seriously questioned (Viskin & Rosso, 2009).

2.2 Studies of the defibrillation threshold

Although successful defibrillations were described in human subject already in the 1940's and 1950's, originally AC current (alternating current) was used for this purpose (Hooker et al, 1933; Beck et al, 1947; Zoll et al, 1956). Gurvich & Yuniev performed in the mid 1930's experiments with DC (direct current) shock defibrillation (Gurvich & Yuniev, 1947). However, this type of defibrillation has become popular only in the early 1960's when Schuder et al published their experiments with truncated direct current shock defibrillation and from then this waveform is used both for clinical and experimental defibrillations (Schuder et al, 1964).

Although, it was known for a long time that the success of defibrillation depends on the shock strength (Hooker et al, 1933), only after the introduction of DC shock defibrillation it has become possible to obtain the above described dose response curve. Different methods were used to increase the delivered energy. Schuder et al used constant-current system to evaluate the defibrillation efficacy and prolonging or shortening the pulse duration they achieved variation in the energy. Latter studies tested the defibrillation by increasing or decreasing the shock energy. In an experimental study, difference of 85±27% in the energy was found between E_{80} and E_{20}, when E_{80} was the energy level with 80% successful defibrillations and similarly E_{20} represents the energy level with 20% successful defibrillations. This study definitely demonstrated the correlation between the shock amplitude and the success of defibrillation (Davy et al, 1987).

The defibrillation energy required for early defibrillation is much lower than after a prolonged episode. The defibrillation energy needed after a few cycles of ventricular fibrillation was 3.0±4.1 Joules and was significantly lower than the energy needed for defibrillation after 10 seconds, which was 15.8±6.6 Joules (Strobel et al, 1998). Prolonged spontaneous or induced ventricular fibrillation, compared to short episodes, required a greater potential gradient for successful defibrillation and to achieve this gradient there was need of higher shock energy (Niemann et al, 2010). After 6 minutes of ventricular fibrillation, the first shock defibrillated the heart in 82% of the cases with 360 Joules biphasic shocks and only in 25% of the cases with 150 Joules biphasic shocks (Walcott et al, 2010). There are several clinical conditions, which require higher than usual energy for successful defibrillation: hypertrophic cardiomyopathy, acute ischemia, and several antiarrhythmic agents. The dose response curve will move rightward in a case of higher defibrillation threshold and to the left with lower defibrillation threshold (Figure 2.4). In the clinical evaluation, if the measured threshold will be higher, also the programmed energy has to be higher to achieve high defibrillation success rate.

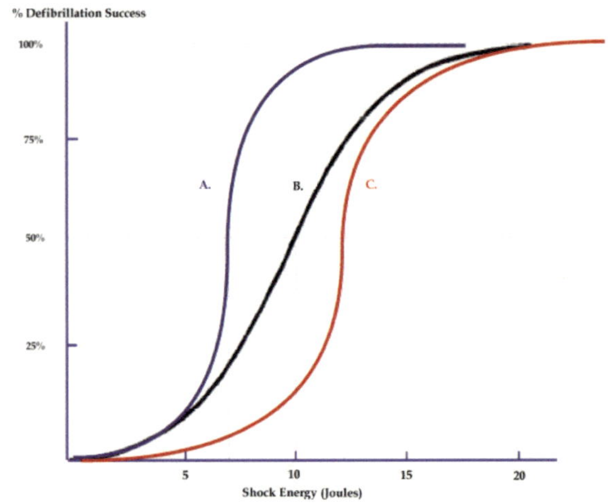

Fig. 2.4. The graph shows 3 dose response curves with different ED_{50} and different pattern. The clinical DFT will be lower in A and highest in C.

2.3 The upper and lower limits of vulnerability

The first requirement for a successful defibrillation is to terminate the fibrillatory activity in the myocardium. However, although the fibrillation may be terminated by the shock, the same shock may reinitiate the fibrillation. Early studies showed than a shock delivered during a vulnerable period may induce ventricular fibrillation (Wiggers & Wegria, 1940). Figure 2.5 shows 2 examples of ventricular fibrillation induction with a shock delivered during the vulnerable period.

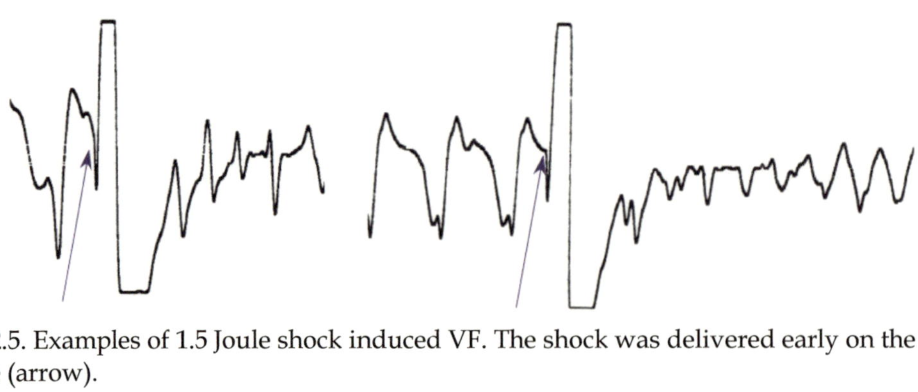

Fig. 2.5. Examples of 1.5 Joule shock induced VF. The shock was delivered early on the T wave (arrow).

Chen at all demonstrated that a shock may induce ventricular fibrillation if it is higher than a certain energy called lower limit of vulnerability and is lower than the upper limit of vulnerability (Chen at al, 1986). Above the upper limit of vulnerability a shock, at any timing, will not induce fibrillation. Interestingly, there was a strong correlation between the upper limit of vulnerability and the defibrillation threshold (Chen at al, 1986; Schauerte, 1999). To avoid reinduction of fibrillation, the defibrillation shock has to be high enough to be above the upper limit of the vulnerability. During experimental defibrillations, different mapping methods resulted in disagreement on the process of defibrillation (Witkowski et al, 1990; Chen et al, 1990; Daubert et al, 1991; Dillon, 1992; Kwaku & Dillon, 1996). However, experimental and simulation methods strongly suggest the re-induction model of defibrillation failure. This re-excitation is avoided if the shock energy is above the upper limit of the vulnerability. Adopted from the brady-pacing area, also defibrillation shocks may generate virtual electrodes. Experimental studies demonstrated that shock might induce virtual electrodes (Kinsley et al, 1994; Wikswo JP et al, 1995; Fast et al, 2002; Sharifov et al, 2004). The picture was completed with the computer simulation methods (Efimov et al, 1997; Efimov et al. 1998; Cheng et al, 1999; Efimov et al, 2000a; Efimov 2000b; Zemlin et al, 2006). Virtual electrode can create singularity points by closing an electrical circle through electrically conducting tissue. Above the upper limit of vulnerability, the shock amplitude is high enough to create opposing electrical poles enough far to impair closure of the circle. A second possibility is that a strong shock will prolong the refractoriness in a large mass of myocardium and this will prevents the closure of the circle. The third possibility is that a successful shock, although terminates the arrhythmia with the virtual electrode mechanism, but being strong enough, will abolish phase singularity point generated by the virtual electrode (Efimov et al, 200b; Trayanova N & Eason, 2002; Trayanova N et al, 2006; Hayashi et al, 2007).

In conclusion, the shock amplitude may contribute to abolishing the fibrillating activity in a large myocardial mass and as a consequence all the fibrillation activity will be terminated. If the shock energy is above the upper limit of vulnerability re-excitation of the already recovered myocardial tissue will be prevented. At the tissue level, the shock abolishes the fibrillation activity; generated virtual electrodes-induced phase singularity, but if the shock is strong enough the singularities vanish before reentry wave generated by them will complete a full circle. As of today, the shock amplitude is the only parameter that can be controlled during defibrillation in both external and internal defibrillators.

3. Shock location and clinical applications of shock vector

Different electrode-pairs can record simultaneously both small and large ventricular fibrillation electrograms (Jones & Klein, 1984). Figure 3.1 shows an example of ventricular fibrillation electrogram with simultaneously recording of low and high amplitude with different electrode-pairs.

Other experimental studies suggested that defibrillation synchronized to high amplitude ventricular fibrillation recording has a higher probability to be successful compared to shocks delivered on low amplitude recordings (Kuelz et al, 1994; Jones at al, 1997). Waveform analysis of ventricular fibrillation electrogram may predict the outcome of the defibrillation (Callaway & Menegazzi, 2005). However, the reason may be the duration of the fibrillation. During early ventricular fibrillation the electrogram is course and the amplitude is high. The cycle length is also longer than during prolonged episode of ventricular fibrillation. As previously mentioned, the energy required to defibrillate the

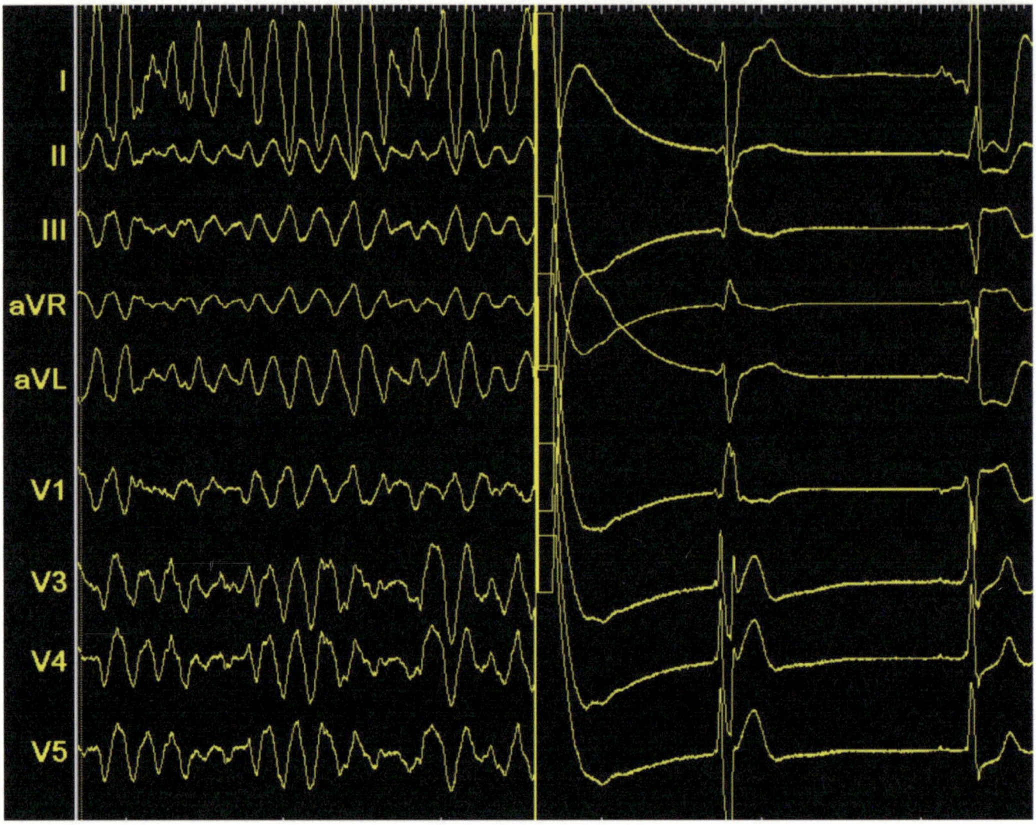

Fig. 3.1. Ventricular fibrillation electrogram showing simultaneously low and high amplitude recording in different leads. The shock terminates the fibrillation and sinus is regained. The amplitude in L_1 is high and at the same time in AVR is low.

heart is much smaller during short duration ventricular fibrillation then after prolonged episodes (Section 2.2).

Brooks et al demonstrated that a shock delivered in a certain direction, chosen because there was high electrogram amplitude on it, was 5-9 times more likely to be successful than other direction without high electrogram amplitude (Brooks et al, 2009). In their study, two shock directions were used: orthogonal and lateral. Using the lateral vector, defibrillation with 30 Joules was more effective than the orthogonal vector, but the difference did not achieve statistical significance. With 50 Joules, in the lateral direction, the success rate was 68.3% (50.2-81.1%) and in the orthogonal direction the success rate was only 18.9% (8.3-37.5%). This difference was statistically significant. When 100 Joules was used the success rate was high and similar with the two vectors, suggesting that a strong shock is successful in any direction (see Section 2.3).

In our study, performed in 20 patients (age 59±12 years, 16 patients with coronary artery disease, left ventricular ejection fraction 0.39±0.08), during defibrillator implantation, 80 defibrillations were performed using monophasic shocks (Rosenheck et al, 2006). The defibrillation shock energy was in the defibrillation threshold zone or immediately below it. The ventricular fibrillation waveform amplitude was 9.5±7.7 mV in the successful attempts and 6.1±4.4mV in the failed attempts (p=0.0318). The monphasic shock has two components on the surface electrogram. A third and large component belongs to the polarization effect. One component is in the same direction with the wavefront direction and the other component is in the opposite direction. We defined the component in the wavefront direction as component 1 and the other one as component 2. Component 1 was divided with component 2. The mean fraction was 0.9±2.2 in the successful defibrillations and 3.2±5.6 in the failed defibrillations (p=0.0006). This is suggesting that the combined shock vector is in the opposite direction to the last fibrillation waveform in the successful attempts and in the direction of the waveform in the failed attempts (Figure 3.2).

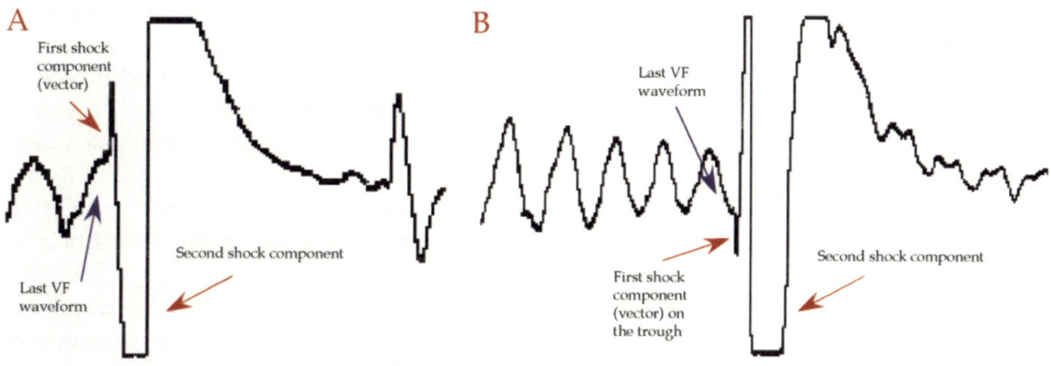

Fig. 3.2. Monophasic shock components and the wavefront direction. The first two components belong to the shock. The third component is the polarization. In picture A, successful defibrillation, the first component in the direction of the waveform (component 1) is significantly smaller then the component against the waveform (component 2) and the 1:2 < 1. In picture B, failed defibrillation, the first component (component 2) is against the waveform direction and 1:2> 1.

4. Shock timing – Basic research

As described in the Section 2.1, the success of defibrillation is correlated to the shock energy in a probabilistic mode, and is described by a dose-response curve. The immediate meaning of this non-linear function is that even at a low energy a small percent of attempts will be successful and during the same time a small percent of the defibrillation attempts at high energy may not be successful. The single logical reason is that the success of defibrillation, although it is possible only with strong shocks, it is also determined by the state of the tissue immediately before the shock.

In an isolated cell the shock will affect the membrane potential and the effect drops over the cell length. It is maximal at the site of the shock and minimal at the opposite site. This decay in the effect at the cellular level is still linear. The major effect is on the extracellular voltage and the effect on the membrane is the difference between the extracellular voltage changes versus the minimal change in the intracellular voltage. Two factors will determine the effect of a shock on the cellular membrane potential, the state of the cell at the moment of the shock and the strength of the stimulus (Drosdall et al, 2010).

At the level of a tissue strand, the effect of the shock will be much more complex. If a non-conducting obstacle will be on the way of the electrical field, which is usually the case, the shock will depolarize as expected the area before the obstacle and will hyperpolarize the area after the obstacle. Due to the difference in the polarity, a current flow will be generated through non-refractory tissue and in a larger three-dimensional tissue wedge fibrillation may be re-induced. A weak shock will have an almost linear effect when a stronger shock has a non-linear effect. Shock may induce also an asymmetric effect with non-equal negative and positive charges in membrane potential. Drosdall et al recently summarized this subject (Drosdall et al, 2010).

In the animal or human heart in situ, the ECG will be the only information on the tissue state during ventricular fibrillation. Therefore, synchronizing the shock to the ECG will affect the outcome of defibrillation. However, the early experiments had controversial data. First of all, the reason for this controversy is the type of ECG used. Using lead L_2, for instance, will describe the electrical state of the myocardium from an angle on the inferior-diaphragmatic wall. This may not be the most representative area for the 3 dimensional tissues.

Other experimental studies evaluated the defibrillation outcome correlated to the amplitude and coarseness of the ECG recording. This may suggest that a large mass of myocardium was depolarized during the shock, meaning that the shock was delivered during the plateau of the action potential in a significant number of cells. However, it is well known that in different leads, during the fibrillation the amplitude may be even opposite. For this reason, not committed recording is needed. In the late studies with implantable defibrillators, the can-to-RV coil electrogram was used, or, as wee will see, in our human study antero-posterior patch-to-patch recording was used.

4.1 Systematic review of the experimental studies

Hsia and Mahmud for the first time evaluated if the random variation in the VF amplitude will affect the success of ventricular defibrillation (Hsia PW & Mahmud R, 1990). The study was performed in 16 dogs. They recorded L_2 electrograms and patch-to-patch recordings. The 50% success energy was determined and in the majority of the dogs it was below 500 V (except 2 dogs with 550 and 600 V, respectively). A total of 82 attempts were successful and 95 failed. The mean defibrillation energy in the successful defibrillations was 6.1±1.4 Joules compared to a similar energy in the failed attempts, 6.2±1.2 Joules. The shock impedance was also similar and only the VF amplitude was significantly higher in the successful defibrillations compared to the failed attempts, 0.5±0.06 mV versus 0.3±0.04 mV. The authors suggested that the cell may be in a relative refractory period during the shock and minimal differences in the shock timing may cause significant changes in the required effective defibrillation energy. A large electrogram may suggest a more advanced synchronization between the electrical sate of the fibrillating myocardial cells. Four examples of defibrillations are provided in the manuscript, two successful and two failed defibrillations. Although the amplitude in the successful examples was higher than in the failed attempts, in the successful defibrillations the shocks are delivered on the upslope and in the failed defibrillations the shocks are delivered on the downslope.

In a second study, moving average was computed on the ventricular fibrillation waveform (Kuelz et al, 1994). Lead L_2 was used for recording. Averages for different length of moving points were calculated and windows from 1-16 provided the best discrimination between successful and failed defibrillation attempts (p between 0.0007 to 0.0022). Above 16, the discriminating power of being course was less. Although these studies suggested the importance of the synchronization between the ventricular fibrillation waveform and the defibrillation shock, no difference between course and fine VF could be shown (Jonse DL & Klein GJ, 1984). They also approved that fine and course ECG recording could be observed simultaneously in different limb leads or chest leads.

Hsia and his collogues, developed a method to detect peak higher than a threshold line (Hsia et al, 1996). If the shock was synchronized to these above-threshold peaks, the success rate was higher by 24%. However, using this method the shock is delivered on the peak of the electrogram. This may suggest that timing might be more important than the recorded amplitude.

The next study was performed in 8 pigs and directly evaluated if shock timing may affect the defibrillation outcome (Hsu et al, 1997). There was no difference in the success between shocks delivered on high or low amplitude electrograms (48% in amplitudes>1.3 mV and 46% in amplitudes<1.3 mV). However, shock delivered on the upslope resulted in 67% success rate and shocks delivered on the downslope resulted only in 39% success rate. The ICD morphology lead was used for recording, with the right ventricular coil as the cathode and the superior vena cava coil and sub-cutaneous array as the anode. Only course electrograms could be analyzed. The conclusion of this study was that timing to upslope, rather than to ECG amplitude is associated with defibrillation success.

Jones et al evaluated if shock synchronized to the action potential from low intensity area would predict favorable outcome of the defibrillation. This study was performed using 6 excised and Langendorff-perfused rabbit hearts. The VF inducing electrodes were placed in the right ventricle, or in the left ventricle. With this method, the basal septum was a low-intensity area and was chosen for monophasic action potential recording (Jones et al, 1997). The shocks were delivered early on the action potential, 5-40% from the start, or late, 40-95%. The energy with 50% chance of defibrillation was determined at both timing (I_{50}). I_{50} decreased by 17% by moving the shock from the late timing to the early timing, 1.48±0.47 mA compared to 1.23±0.21 mA. This 17% reduction in the current corresponds to 31% reduction in the energy. The dose-response curve of the early shocks was displaced to the left with a narrow standard deviation (see Figure 2.4 for explanation).

In a prospective study, Hsu at al developed software synchronizing the shock to four different parts of the VF waveform, as recorded with an ICD morphology electrogram (Hsu et al, 1998). The peak (maximal amplitude) and trough (minimum amplitude) were defined. The upslope was divided into three timings. Only high-amplitude recordings were used. The synchronized defibrillations were compared with random defibrillations. The dose-response curve of probability-of-success versus shock intensity moved to left with the synchronized shock versus the random shocks (see Figure 2.4 for explanation). The E_{80} (energy with expected 80% success of defibrillation) decreased significantly from 27.1±2.5 Joules to 22.9±1.8 Joules. This study suggests, that shock synchronized to the upslope on the morphology electrogram of an implantable defibrillator, in an animal model, improved the defibrillation efficacy. Therefore, both the retrospective and the prospective experimental studies demonstrated that synchronizing the shock to the upslope of a noncommited electrogram, in this case the morphology electrogram, improves the defibrillation. Parallel, shocks synchronized to the early part of the action potential also improved the defibrillation. For this reason, the upslope may represent the early segment of the action potential and the downslope the late segment. All this studies evaluate the defibrillation in short induced episodes of ventricular fibrillation, not exciding 20 seconds and the relevance of their conclusions is limited.

4.2 Defibrillation of prolonged episodes of ventricular fibrillation

As of today, a new area in the world of defibrillation is evolving, the automatic external defibrillators. As opposed to the conventional external defibrillators the automatic defibrillators requires preprogramming of the energy, just like the implantable devices. The use of these external automatic defibrillators will be necessarily later than 10-15 seconds. Therefore, additional studies are needed to evaluate the importance of timing in prolonged episodes of ventricular fibrillation termination. Several studies evaluated the ventricular fibrillation electrogram amplitude spectral area (AMSA) and slope not to predict merely the defibrillation efficacy, but to predict the result of resuscitation (Indik et al, 2010; Povoas & Bisera 2000). As previously mentioned (Section 3), the high waveform amplitude may suggest short duration ventricular fibrillation and not necessarily timing. Obviously the result of resuscitation will be significantly different if performed early than after prolonged episode of ventricular fibrillation. For this reason, further studies on the preshock electrograms in these prolonged episodes of ventricular fibrillation is still needed.

5. Shock timing – Clinical data

Based on the experimental data, we purposed to evaluate the importance of defibrillation shock timing in human subjects during defibrillator implantation or during later defibrillation evaluation. First of all, we were searching for a reproducible and not committed electrogram. As is evident in Figure 5.1 and 5.2 when the fibrillation is recorded simultaneously in different standard ECG leads, the recording may be very different in simultaneously recorded leads. If at a particular time, on L_1, the recording is course, in lead L_2 may be fine. The shock may be on the upslope on L_3 and precordial leads, but on the downslope on L_1 and L_2. The late experimental studies have used the morphology lead ECG (between the ICD can and the RV defibrillation lead, or between the superior vena cava defibrillation coil and the right ventricular defibrillation coil). Our study was performed using two large surface patch electrodes with a general antero-posterior and supero-inferior axis. One of the patch-electrodes was placed on the right side of the chest and the second patch-electrode was placed on the left side of the back. This recording was not committed neither to the antero-posterior axis, nor superior-inferior axis, but was a more general recording combining both directions. Figure 5.2 shows defibrillation on 12-lead ECG and Figure 5.3 the patch-to-patch recording.

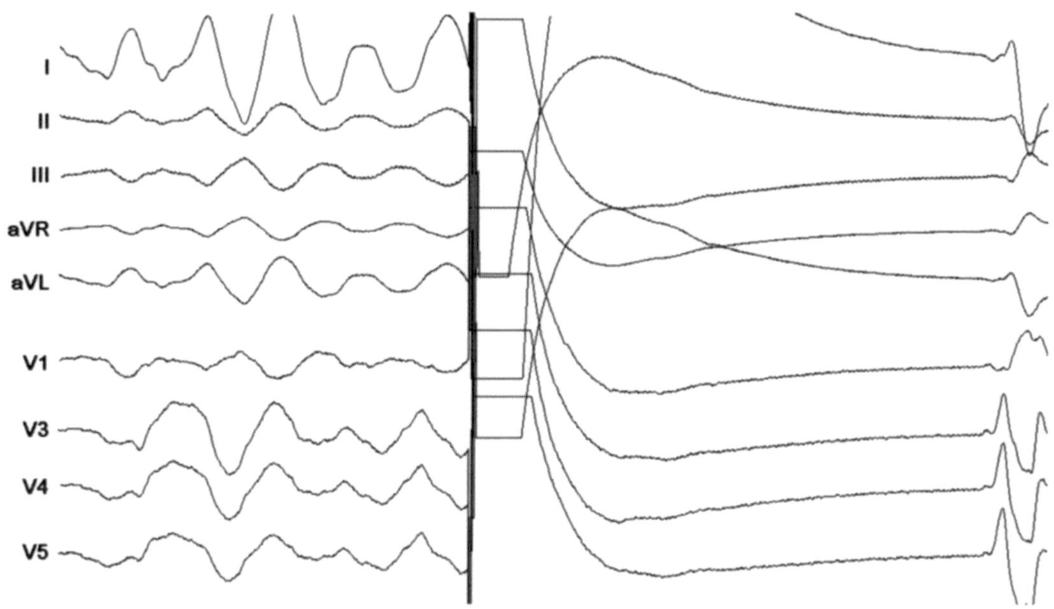

Fig. 5.1. Recording at 100mm/sec, 9 lead ECG of ventricular fibrillation and defibrillation with implantable defibrillator, 14 Joules. The VF amplitude is high in lead 1, V_3 and low in leads 2, 3, V_1.

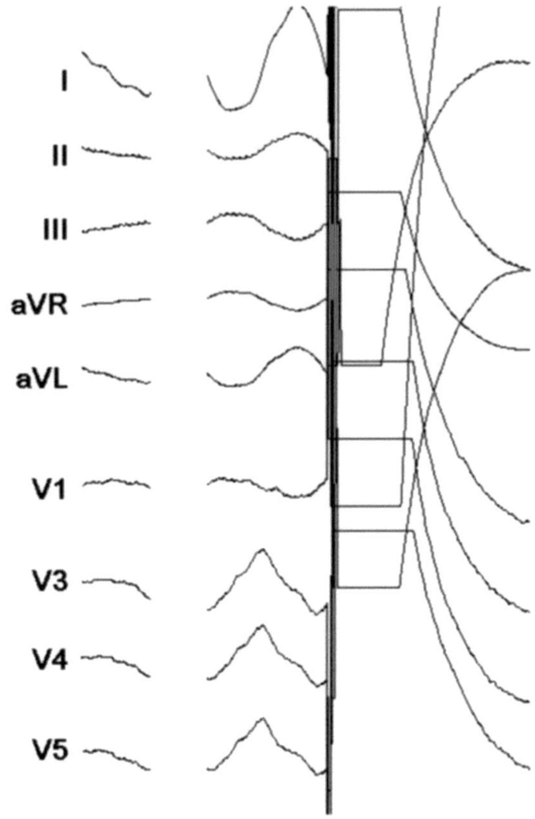

Fig. 5.2. The shock is delivered on the downslope in lead 1, 2, AVL and on upslope on leads 3, V_1, V_3, V_4, V_5.

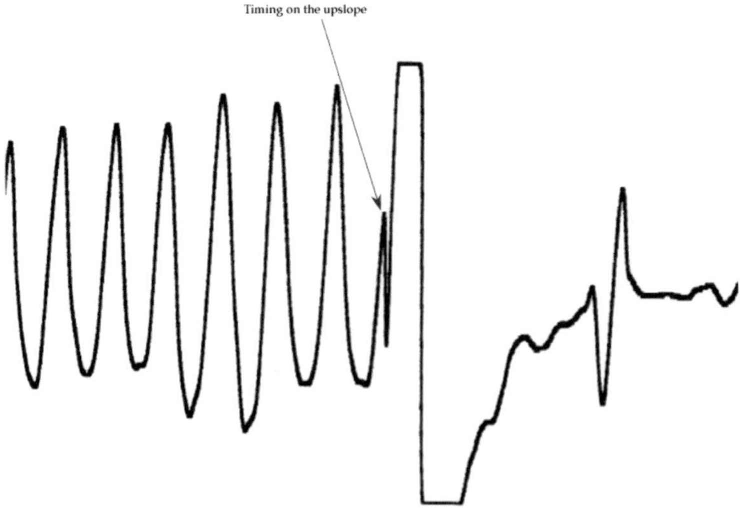

Fig. 5.3. A patch-to-patch recording with clear timing of the shock.

5.1 Shock timing studies in human hearts using biphasic shocks

Our preliminary data was presented during an international symposium on cardiac arrhythmias (9th Congress of the International Society for Holter and Noninvasive Electrocardiology and International Congress on Cardiac Pacing and Electrophysiology, Istanbul, Turkey September 23-27, 2000) and published in a monograph (Rosenheck et al, 2000). The last analysis was presented at the Heart Rhythm Association Annual Meeting in 2005 (Rosenheck & Sharon, 2005). The study is still ongoing.
Figure 5.4 shows the definition of the shock timing on patch-to-patch recording.

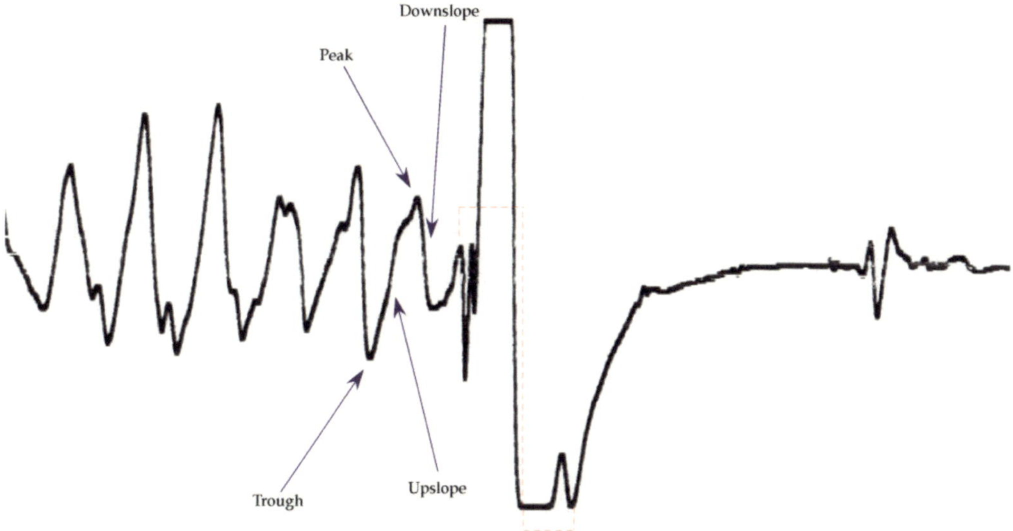

Fig. 5.4. Timing markers: Trough, peak, upslope and downslope. The first shock vector might be very complex like in this case. A single ventricular ectopic beat is evident on the last part of the shock recording (break stimulation).

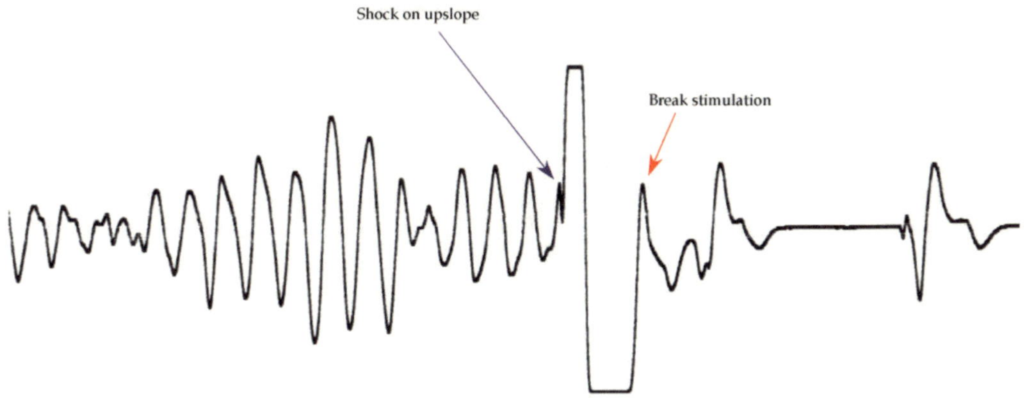

Fig. 5.5. Successful defibrillation with the shock delivered on the upslope. There is a limited post shock ventricular activity starting with the shock end and is suggestive of break stimulation without propagating it as result of prolonged refractoriness.

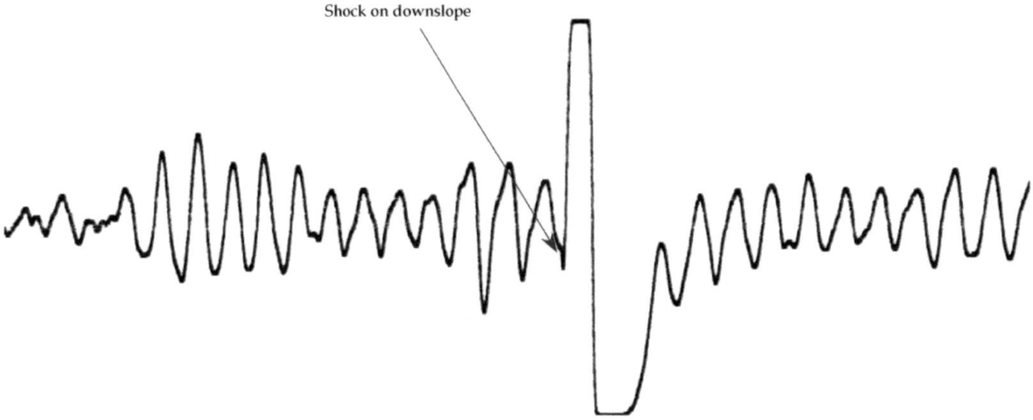

Fig. 5.6. Failed defibrillation with the shock delivered on the downslope. There is a slight difference between the preshock and post shock ventricular fibrillation waveform.

In the first report, 450 episodes of ventricular defibrillation were studied. The patch-to-patch ECG was recoded during ICD implantation and defibrillation evaluation. The electrograms were collected from 110 patients (88 male and 22 women). The mean age was 56±16 years and the majority of the patients had coronary artery disease. The defibrillation effectiveness was evaluated using the Multi-step test (Figure 2.3B). Patients with low defibrillation thresholds were not necessarily studied until failed defibrillation was achieved and the test was discontinued if 6 Joule-shock defibrillated the heart. This was called the best-predicted DFT. Two groups were defined. One group, the outlying group, had either a very low defibrillation threshold or patients with high defibrillation threshold (between 18-25 Joules). Patients with defibrillation threshold > 25 Joules were excluded. In the second group, the mid group, all the attempts were defibrillated with energy between 10-18 Joules. Ninety-four episodes were in the outlying group and 356 in the mid group. In the outlying group, 74.1% of the shocks delivered on the upslope were successful versus 45% of the shocks on the downslope were successful ($p<0.01$). In the mid group the success rate of the defibrillation on both upslope and downslope were similar and above 80%. The conclusion was, that in the outlying group the efficacy was significantly higher on the upslope, because the narrower safety margin between the measured efficacy and the real DFT. In the mid group the safety margin was much wider and this relatively strong defibrillation shock may be effective in any way. Figure 5.5 shows a successful defibrillation on the upslope of the electrogram and Figure 5.6 shows a failed defibrillation on the downslope.

In the second study, 1374 additional episodes were included and studied. On the upslope, 87.3% of the defibrillations were successful and on the downslope 56.7% ($p<0.0001$ and relative risk of failure on the downslope 1.442 [1.414 to 1.682]). In the best-predicted DFT zone 79.7% were on the upslope and in the lower energy group only 57.6 were on upslope ($p<0.001$). This study demonstrated strong association between the shock timing on upslope and success of defibrillation. The duration of the episodes was 8-10 seconds. The patch-to-patch electrogram was coarse with intermittent short episodes of fine VF. The majority of the defibrillation shocks were on the large amplitude electrograms in both successful and failed attempts and the graphic analysis was easily performed.

5.2 Shock timing study in human heart using monophasic shock

Additional information was obtained by analyzing patch-to-patch defibrillation electrograms using monophasic shocks and was presented at the World Congress of Cardiology 2006 (Rosenheck et al, 2006). Monophasic shocks were used in this study, to avoid more complex effect of the biphasic shocks, especially when the vectors are studied. In this study 96 defibrillation attempts with monophasic shocks were evaluated. The antero-posterior vector, the amplitude of VF electrogram and the shock timing were studied. Eighty episodes were defibrillated with energy at the clinical DFT or with immediately lower energy (50 at the DFT and 30 lower energy). In the successful defibrillations 84% were on the upslope and in the failed attempts only 37% were on the upslope ($p<0.01$). As presented in Section 3, the electrogram amplitude and the shock vector direction had also significant effect on the success of defibrillation in these 20 patients (Figure 3.2). In addition to the importance of the timing, information on the underlying electrical activity and the interaction between the dominant VF vector and the shock vector were demonstrated (Section 3).

Although the conclusion after the experimental studies was that early shock might prolong the refractoriness and create conduction blocks in a critical mass of myocardium, more recent hypothesis on the mechanism of defibrillation may be used to explain our clinical results. It is accepted today that a shock has a non-uniform effect on the tissue. Both areas of depolarization and hyperpolarization are generated (Wikswo, 1994; Effimov et al, 1997). Obviously, the presence of both polarities, during the same time, will behave like an electrode, more precisely as a virtual electrode. The inversely polarized areas may be asymmetric, with one of the poles larger than the other. Internal nonconducting obstacles may facilitate this opposite polarization. If these poles are adjacent, a singularity point may be generated and a new spiral wave initiated (Efimov et al, 1998). Early shocks, when a large mass of myocardial cells are in their early phase of action potential, although may generate virtual electrode, but no excitable and conducting tissue will connect between the opposite polarized tissues. Slightly latter shocks may initiate the virtual electrodes and enough tissue may be already recovered to serve as electrical conducting tissue. Two adjacent polarized areas will provide the stimulation electrodes and non-refractory excitable tissue between them will provide the substrate for reentry.

The direction of the shock vector may also be explained with this new hypothesis. If the net shock vector is opposite to the main fibrillation waveform vector, it is less possibility to generate virtual electrode as the tissue is depolarized by the large wavefront. Moreover, a large mass of refractory myocardium will interfere with the conduction between the poles and the electrodes are abolished before the circle can be completed. It is also recently suggested that the main tissue responsible for the reinitiating the post-shock arrhythmia are the Purkinje Cells Network (Deo et al, 2009). These cells are densely distributed in the septum and the same area is also rich in singularity points (Trayanova, 2006). This may also contribute to the understanding of the importance of shock direction.

6. Conclusions and future directions

In addition to the contribution of the shock amplitude to the success of defibrillation, the shock orientation compared to the fibrillation waveform and shock timing is important for the defibrillation outcome. Experimental and clinical studies are supporting the importance of these three shock characteristics in the outcome of ventricular defibrillation. Understanding of these contributors to the defibrillation mechanism is important not only academically but also in the clinical practice. In the era of implantable defibrillators and automatic external defibrillators it is utmost important to understand the determinants of successful defibrillation. Implementing the timing and shock orientation in the defibrillation devices may improve the efficacy and the outcome of the defibrillation both for the implantable devices and non-professional operated external defibrillators.

7. References

Bardy GH, Ivey TD, Allen MD, Johnson G, Mehra R & Green HL. (1989) A prospective evaluation of biphasic versus monophasic pulse on defibrillation efficacy in humans. J Am Coll Cardiol 14:728-733

Bardy GH, Johnson G, Poole JE at al. (1993) A simplified, single-lead unipolar transvenous cardioversion-defibrillation system. Circulation 88:543-547

Beck CS, Pritchard WH & Feil HS. (1947) Ventricular fibrillation of long duration abolished by electric shock. JAMA 135:985-986

Brooks L, Zhang Y, Dendi R, Anderson RH, Zimmerman B & Kerber RE. (2009) Selecting the transthoracic defibrillation shock direction vector based on VF amplitude improves shock success. J Cardiovasc Electrophysiol 20:1032-1038

Callaway CW & Menegazzi JJ. Waveform analysis of ventricular fibrillation to predict defibrillation. (2005) Curr Opin Crit Care 11:192-199

Chen PS, Shibata N, Dixon EG, Martin RO & Ideker RE. (1986) Comparison of the defibrillation threshold and the upper limit of ventricular vulnerability. Circulation 73:1022-1028

Chen PS, Wolf PD, Melnick SD, Danieley ND, Smith WM & Ideker RE. (1990) Comparison of activation during ventricular fibrillation and following unsuccessful defibrillation shock in open-chest dogs. Circ Res 66:1544-1560

Cheng Y, Mowrey KA, Van Wagoner DR, Tchou PJ & Efimov IR. (1999) Virtual electrode - induced reexcitation. A mechanism of defibrillation. Circ Res 85:1056-1066

Dalal D, Nasir K, Bomma C, Prakasa K, Tandri H, Piccini J, Roguin A, Tichnell C, James C, Russell SD, Judge DP, Abraham T, Spevak PJ, Bluemke DA & Calkins H. (2005) Arrhythmogenic right ventricular dysplasia. A United States experience. Circulation 112:3823–3832

Daubert JP, Frazier DW, Wolf PD, Franz MR, Smith WM & Ideker RE. (1991) Response of relative refractory canine myocardium to monophasic and biphasic shock. Circulation 84:2522-2538

Daubert JP, ZarebaW, Rosero SZ, Budzikowski A, Robinson JL & Moss AJ. (2007) Role of implantable cardioverter defibrillator therapy in patients with long QT syndrome. Am Heart J 153:S53–S58

Davy JM, Fain ES, Dorian P & Winkle RA. (1987) The relationship between successful defibrillation and delivered energy in open-chest dogs: Reappraisal of the "defibrillation Threshold" concept. Am Heart J 113:77-84

Deakin CD, Nolan JP, Sunde K &Koster RW. (2010) European resuscitation council guidelines for Resuscitation 2010 section 3: automatic external defibrillators, defibrillation cardioversion and pacing. Resuscitation 81:1293-1304

Deo M, Boylle P, Plank G & Vigmond E. (2009) Arrhythmogenic mechanism of the Purkinje system during electrical shocks: a modeling study. Heart Rhythm 6:1782-1789

Desai AS, Fang JC, Maisel WH & Baughmann KL. (2004) Implantable cardioverter defibrillator for prevention of mortality in patients with nonischemic cardiomyopathy. A meta-analysis of randomized controlled trials. JAMA 292:2874–2879

Dillon SM. (1992) Synchronized repolarization after defibrillation shock. A possible component of the defibrillation process demonstrated by optical recording in rabbit heart. Circulation 85:1865-1878

Drosdall DJ, Fast VG & Ideker RE. (2010) Mechanism of defibrillation. Annu Rev Bimed Eng 12:233-258

Efimov IR, Cheng YA, Biermann M, Van Wagoner DR, Magalev TN & Tchou PJ. (1997) Transmembrane voltage changes produced by real and virtual electrodes during monophasic defibrillation shock delivered by an implantable electrode. J Cardiovasc Electrophysiol 8:1031-1045

Efimov IR, Cheng Y, Van Wagoner DR, Mazgalev T & Tchou PJ. (1998) Virtual electrode-induced phase singularity: a basic mechanism of defibrillation failure. Circ Res 82:918-925

Efimov IR, Aguel F, Cheng Y, Wollenzier B & Trayanova N. (2000a) Virtual electrode depolarization in the far field: implications for external defibrillation. Am J Physiol Circ Physiol 279:H1055-H1070

Efimov IR, Cheng Y, Yamabouchi Y & Tchou PJ. (2000b) Direct evidence of the role of virtual electrode-induced phase singularity in success and failure of defibrillation. J Cardiovasc Electrophysiol 2:861-868

Ezekowitz JA, Amstrong PW & McAlister FA. (2003) Implantable cardioverter defibrillator in primary and secondary prevention: a systematic review of randomized, controlled trials. Ann Intern Med 138:445–452

Fast VG, Sharifov OF, Cheek ER, Newton JC & Ideker RE. (2002) Intramural virtual electrodes during defibrillation shocks in left ventricular wall assessed by optical mapping of membrane potential. Circulation 106:1007-1014

Folke F, Gislason GH, Lippert FK, Nielsen SL, Weeke P, Hansen ML, Fosbol EL, Andersen SS, Rasmussen S, Schramm TK, Kober L & Torp-Pedersen C. (2010) Differences between out-of-hospital cardiac arrest in residential and public locations and implications for public-access defibrillation. Circulation 122:623-630

Gurvich NL, & Yuniev GS. Restoration of heart rhythm during fibrillation by a condenser discharge. (1947) Am Rev Soviet Med 4:252-256

Hayashi H, Lin SF & Chen PS. (2007) Preshock phase singularity and the outcome of ventricular defibrillation. Heart Rhythm 4:927-934

Higgins S, Mann D, Calkins H, Estes MNA, Strickberger SA, Breiter D, Lang D & Hahn S. (2005) One conversion of ventricular fibrillation is adequate for implantable cardioverter-defibrillator implant: An analysis from the Low Energy Safety Study (LESS). Heart Rhythm 2:117-122

Hooker DR, Kouwenhoven WB & Langworthy OR. The effect of alternating currents on the heart. (1933) Am J Physiol 103:444-454

Hsia PW & Mahmud R. (1990) Genesis of sigmoidal dose-response curve during defibrillation by random shocks: a theoretical model based on experimental evidence for a vulnerable window during ventricular fibrillation. Pacing Clin Electrophysiol 13:1326-1342

Hsia PW, Freck S, Allen CA, Wise RM, Cohen NM & Damiano RJ. (1996) A critical period of ventricular fibrillation more susceptible to defibrillate: real-time waveform analysis using single ECG lead. Pacing Clin Electrophysiol 19:418-430

Hsu W, Lin Y, Heil JE, Jones J & Lang DJ. (1997) Effect of shock timing on defibrillation success. Pacing Clin Electrophysiol 20:153-157

Hsu W, Lin Y, Lang DJ & Jones JL. (1998) Improved internal defibrillation success with shocks timed to morphology electrograms. Circulation 98:808-812

Huikuri HV, Castellanos A & Myerburg RJ. (2001) Sudden cardiac death due to cardiac arrhythmias. N Engl J Med 345:1475-1482

Indik JH, Allen D, Shanmugasundaram M, Zuercher M, Hilwig RW, Berg RA & Kern KB. (2010) Predictors of resuscitation in swine model of ischemic and nonischemic ventricular fibrillation cardiac arrest: Superiority of amplitude spectral area and slope to predict a return of spontaneous circulation when resuscitation efforts are prolonged. Crit Care Med 38:2352-2357

Jacobs I, Sunde K, Deakin CD, Hazinski MF, Kerber RE, Koster RW, Morrison LJ, Nolan JP, Sayre MR & Defibrillation Chapter Collaborators. (2010) Part 6: Defibrillation: 2010 International consensus on cardiopulmonary resuscitation and emergency cardiovascular care science with treatment recommendation. Circulation 122:S325-S337

Jonse DL & Klein GJ. (1984) Ventricular fibrillation: the importance of being course? J Electrocardiol 17:393-400

Jones DL. Irish WD & Klein GJ. (1991) Defibrillation Efficacy; Comparison of the defibrillation threshold versus dose-response curve determination. Circ Res 69:45-51

Jones JL, Noe WA, Moulder C, Tovar OH, Hsu W & Lin Y. (1997) Synchronized shock reduce defibrillation threshold. Proceedings-19th International Conference-IEEE/EMBS 145-147

Kwaku KF & Dillon SM. (1996) Shock-induced depolarization of refractory myocardium prevents wave –front propagation in defibrillation. Circ Res 79:957-973

Kinsley SB, Hill BC & Ideker RE. (1994) Virtual electrode effect in myocardial fibers. Biophys J. 66:719-728

Kitamura T, Iwami T, Kawamura T, Nagao K, Tanaka H & Hiraide A. (2010) Nationwide public-access defibrillation in Japan. N Engl J Med 362:994-1004

Knecht S, Sacher F, Wight M, Hocini M, Nogami A, Arentz T, Petit B, Franck R, De Chillou C, Lamaoson D, Farre J, Lavergne T, Verbeet T, Nault I, Matsou S, Leroux L. Weerasooriya R, Cauchemez B, Lellouche N, Derval N, Narayan SM, Jais P, Clementy J & Haissahuerre M. (2009) Long-term follow-up of idiopathic ventricular fibrillation ablation: a multicenter study. J Am Coll Cardiol 54:522-528

Kuelz KW, Hsia PW, Wise RM, Mahmud R & Damiano RJ. (1994) Integration of absolute ventricular fibrillation voltage with successful defibrillation. IEEE Transaction Biomed Eng 41:782-790

Maron BJ. (2000) Hypertrophic cardiomyopathy. A systematic review. JAMA 287:1308–1320

Niemann JT, Rosborough JP, Youngquist ST & Shah AP. (2010) Transthoracic defibrillation potential gradients in a closed chest porcine model of prolonged spontaneous and electrical induced ventricular fibrillation. Resuscitation 81:447-480

Povoas HP & Bisera J. (2000) Electrocardiographic waveform analysis for predicting success of defibrillation. Crit Care Med 11 (Suppl.):N210-N211

Rea TD, Olsufka M, Bemis B, White L, Yin L, Becker L, Copass M, Eisenberg M & Cobb L. (2010) A population-based investigation of public access defibrillation: role of emergency medical services care. Resuscitation 81:163-167

Rho RW, Page RL. (2011) Public access defibrillation. Heart Fail Clin A7:269-276

Rosenheck S, Leibowitz D & Sharon Z. (2000) The effect of shock timing on the ventricular defibrillation in human hearts. In Oto A ed. New Trends in Electrocardiology. Monduzzi Editore, Bologna, Italy 107-112

Rosenheck S & Sharon Z. (2005) Shock timing on the upslope of the fibrillation electrogram improves the defibrillation success. Heart Rhythm 2 (Supp):S85-S86

Rosenheck S, Weiss A & Sharon Z. (2006) Shock timing, amplitude and underlying electrical activity determine success of defibrillation in humans using monophasic shocks. Eur Heart J 27 (suppl 1):468

Rosenheck S, Gorni S, Katz I, Rabin A, Shpoliansky U, Mandelbaum M & Weiss AT. (2009a) Modified alternating current defibrillation-A new defibrillation technique. Europace 11:239-244

Rosenheck S, Sharon Z & Weiss A. (2009b) Long-term follow-up of patients with relatively high effective defibrillation threshold during cardioverter defibrillator implantation with endocardial leads. Cardiology 112:107-113

Rosenheck S, Weiss A & Sharon Z. (2010) Therapy success and survival in patients with valvular heart disease and Implantable Cardioverter Defibrillator. Int J Cardiol 144:103-104

Sacher F, Probst V, Iesaka Y, Jacon P, Laborderie J, Mizon-Gérard F, MaboP, Reuter S, Lamaison D, Takahashi Y, O'Neill MD, Garrigue S, Pierre B, Jaïs P, Pasquié JL, Hocini M, Salvador-Mazenq M, Nogami A, Amiel A, Defaye P, Bordachar P, BovedaS, Maury P, Klug D, Babuty D, Haïssaguerre M, Mansourati J, Clémenty J, & Le Marec H. (2006) Outcome after implantation of cardioverter-defibrillator in patients with Brugada syndrome. A multicenter study. Circulation 114:2317–2324

Sharifov OF, Ideker RE & Fast VG. (2004) High-resolution optical mapping of intramural virtual electrodes in porcine left ventricular wall. Cardiovasc Res 64:448-456

Schauerte PN, Ziegert K, Waldmann M, Schondube FA, Birkenhauer F, Mischke K, Grossmann M, Hanrath P & Stelbrink C. (1999) Effect of biphasic shock duration on defibrillation threshold with different electrode configuration and phase 2-capacitance. Prediction by upper-limit-of-vulnerability determination. Circulation 99:1516-1522

Silka MJ & Bar-Cohen Y. (2006) Pacemaker and implantable cardioverter defibrillators in pediatric patients. Heart Rhythm 3:1360–1366

Schuder JC, Stoeckle H & Dolan AM. (1664) Transthoracic ventricular defibrillation with square-wave stimuli: one-half cycle, one cycle, and multicycle waveforms. Circ Res 15:258-264

Strobel JS, Kenknight BH, Rollins DL, Smith WM & Ideker RE. (1998) The effect of ventricular fibrillation duration and site of induction on the defibrillation threshold during early ventricular fibrillation. J Am Coll Cardiol 32:521-527

Trayanova N & Eason J. (2002) Shock induced arrhythmogenesis in the myocardium. Chaos 12:962-971

Trayanova N. (2006) Defibrillation of the heart: insights into mechanisms from modeling studies. Exp Physiol 91:323-337

Trayanova N, Plank G & Rodriguez B. (2006) What we have learned from mathematical models of defibrillation and postshock arrhythmogenesis? Application of bidomaine simulation. Heart Rhythm 3:1232-1235

Viskin S & Rosso R. (2008) The top 10 reasons to avoid defibrillation testing during ICD implantation. Heart Rhythm 5:391-393

Walcott GP, Melnick SB, Killingsworth CR & Ideker RE. (2010) Comparison of low-energy versus high-energy biphasic defibrillation shocks following prolonged ventricular fibrillation. Prehospital Emergency Care 14:62-70

Wiggers CJ. (1940) The physiologic basis for cardiac resuscitation from ventricular fibrillation-methods for serial defibrillation. Am Heart J 20:413-422

WiggersCJ & Wegria R. (1940) Ventricular fibrillation due to single localized induction and condenser shock applied during the vulnerable phase of the ventricular systole. Am Heart J 20:500-505

Wikswo JP. (1994) The complexity of cardiac cables: Virtual electrode effect. Biophysical J 66:551-553

Wikswo JP, Lin SF, Abbas RA. (1995) Virtual electrodes in cardiac tissue; a common mechanism for anodal and cathodal stimulation. Biophys J. 69:2195-2210

Winkle RA. (2010) The effectiveness and cost effectiveness of public-access defibrillation. Clin Cardiol 3:396-399

Witkowski FX, Penkoske PA & Plonsey R. (1990) Mecahnism of cardiac defibrillation in open-chest dogs with unipolar DC-coupled simultaneous activation and shock potential recording. Circulation 82:244-260

Zemlin CW, Mironov S & Pertsov AM. (2006) Near-threshold field stimulation; Intramural versus surface activity. Cardiovasc Res 69:98-106

Zipes DP, Fischer J, King RM, Nicoll A deB & Jolly WW. (1975) Termination of ventricular fibrillation in dogs by depolarizing a critical amount of myocardium. Am J Cardiol 36:37-44

Zoll PM, Linenthal AJ, Gibson W, Paul MH & Norman LR. (1956) Termination of ventricular fibrillation in man by externally applied electrical countershock. N Engl Med 254:727-732

3

Prognostic Significance of Implantable Cardioverter-Defibrillator Shocks

Dan Blendea[1], Razvan Dadu[2] and Craig McPherson[2]
[1]*Massachusetts General Hospital - Harvard Medical School*
[2]*Bridgeport Hospital – Yale University School of Medicine*
United States of America

1. Introduction

Therapy with implantable cardioverter-defibrillators (ICDs) has been shown to improve survival among several large groups of patients at risk for sudden cardiac death (SCD). Several complicating issues arose from the widespread use of ICDs especially in heart failure (HF) patients. Twenty percent to 35% of HF patients who receive an ICD for primary prevention of SCD will receive an appropriate shock within 1 to 3 years for a life-threatening arrhythmia.[1] Almost half of the HF patients who survive a cardiac arrest and receive an ICD for secondary prevention will receive a shock within 1 year of implant.[2] Implantable cardioverter-defibrillator (ICD) shocks are usually regarded with a sense of relief given that the ventricular tachyarrhythmia was treated, and the SCD was averted. There is, however, accumulating data from the literature showing that patients with ICDs who receive shocks, whether appropriate or spurious, have worse prognosis than similar patients who do not receive shocks.

Current guidelines do not provide a clear approach to managing patients presenting with ICD shocks, who clearly represent a high-risk group. However, current data from the literature suggest that ICD shocks should prompt a thorough evaluation to determine the etiology of the shock and to help guide therapeutic interventions.

2. Initial evaluation after ICD discharge

The initial evaluation of the patient who receives an ICD shock begins with interrogation of the device. The timing of the device interrogation depends on the number of shocks and related symptoms.[3] In case of an isolated shock without change in clinical status or symptoms, evaluation should generally occur within a few days.[4] Multiple ICD shocks or shocks associated with worsening HF symptoms, syncope, angina, or electrical storm warrant emergent medical attention.[4]

Device interrogation will reveal whether the ICD shock was appropriate or inappropriate. While there is still some debate regarding the definition of an appropriate shock, most authors agree that any shock for ventricular tachycardia (VT) or ventricular fibrillation (VF) is considered appropriate.

The acute management strategies depend on the specific etiology of the shock. If the shock was appropriate the next step is to address reversible causes, check and correct electrolytes, consider antiarrhythmic therapy, optimize betablocker treatment, optimize device therapies including antitachycardia pacing (ATP), and consider intubation and sedation for refractory VT or VF. If the shock was inappropriate the acute strategy is to treat the supraventricular tachycardia, optimize device programming, and assess for possible lead oversensing.[3]

In addition to all these acute management strategies it is important to realize that even though the SCD might have been prevented by the ICD shock, the natural history of the disease is now transformed and there is accumulating data suggesting that the prognosis of the group of patients who receive shocks, especially in HF patients, is worse than the rest of the ICD patients.

3. Appropriate ICD shocks

3.1 Prognostic importance of appropriate ICD shocks

Several large trials have shown that therapy with ICDs improves survival among patients who are at risk for SCD.[3, 5, 6] Based on these results the implantation of an ICD for primary prevention has become standard of care for patients who meet the high-risk criteria.[7] One potential result of the broader use of ICDs is that the natural history of the disease in these patients is modified as a consequence of the delivery of ICD therapies. The results of the MADIT II were the first to demonstrate an adverse prognosis associated with ICD therapy used for primary prevention.[8, 9] In this study, among 719 patients with ischemic heart disease, an ICD shock or antitachycardia pacing was reported to be appropriate in 23.5%. The risk of death, was found to be increased by a factor of more than 3 among patients who received ICD shocks or antitachycardia pacing for ventricular tachycardia or ventricular fibrillation.[8]

After an ICD shock for a life-threatening arrhythmia, hospitalizations for HF were more frequent, and mortality was increased 3-fold.[10] Within one year of an ICD shock for ventricular tachycardia (VT) or ventricular fibrillation (VF), the probability of an HF event was 26% and 31%, respectively, while it was 19% for those not having an ICD.[10] The corresponding survival rate one year after initial ICD shock for VT or VF was 80% and the survival curves were related to the rate of the presenting tachycardia. Increased tachycardia rates were associated with lower survival rates. Other clinical factors associated with increased mortality after appropriate ICD discharge, were blood urea nitrogen, lack of beta-blockade, NYHA functional class, presence of atrial fibrillation (AF), and diabetes mellitus.[10] The ICD therapy was associated with a 39% increased risk of a first HF hospitalization and a 58% increase in recurrent admission for HF.[10]

Analysis of data from the Sudden Cardiac Death in Heart Failure Trial (SCD-HeFT)[1] showed findings consistent with those of the MADIT-II study.[3] In the SCD-HeFT study, 33% of HF patients received an ICD shock. Among these patients treated with ICD discharges the most common cause of death was progressive HF. Patients receiving an appropriate shock had a 5-fold increase in risk of death, whereas patients receiving an inappropriate shock had a 2-fold increase in risk of death. Multiple shocks increased the risk of death more than single shocks. The median time from shock to death was 168 days among patients receiving appropriate shocks and 294 days among patients receiving inappropriate shocks.[3]

The risk of death with appropriate ICD shocks was higher in the study by Poole et al. [1] - increased by a factor of more than 5. The higher risk of death associated with appropriate ICD shocks found by Poole and colleagues in comparison to the MADIT II study may be related to the longer follow-up and the exclusion of patients with NYHA class I disease (selection of patients with higher risk than those in MADIT II). In addition these results reflect the use of primarily single-lead ICDs, a single zone of therapy, and shock-only programming for high-rate arrhythmias that were most likely to be life-threatening.[1] Similar to MADIT-II patients, SCD-HeFT patients with NYHA functional class III and ischemic cardiomyopathy had a shorter duration between initial shock and death. Subgroup analyses from MADIT-II trial confirm that ICD shocks increase the risk for first and recurrent HF events.[2, 10]

One of the most important questions generated by these results is why ICD patients tend to have worsening prognosis and more frequent HF after an ICD shock. Myocardial damage induced by ICD shocks may contribute to worsening HF.[11, 12] This is suggested by the adverse impact on prognosis of inappropriate shocks. In the MADIT-II study, however, inappropriate shocks did not increase the risk of adverse outcomes. In the study by Poole and colleagues, mortality after an inappropriate shock was approximately 3-fold less than after appropriate therapy, thus downplaying the role of shock-induced myocardial damage contributing to HF risk, and suggesting that arrhythmia may simply be a marker of worsening HF.[3]

In an editorial comment on the study of Poole et al., Healey and Connolly surmised the situation as follows: "Although it is plausible that shocks somehow have an adverse effect on myocardial function, this is unlikely to be a major factor. What is much more likely is that the occurrence of a ventricular arrhythmia that causes a shock is signaling a meaningful change in the patient's clinical status….occurrence of shocks is not a random event in an otherwise stable clinical course but a sign of clinical deterioration in the underlying disease process."[44] We concur with this opinion. Furthermore, inappropriate ICD discharges, which largely result from atrial fibrillation or other rapidly conducting supraventricular tachycardias may be associated with higher subsequent mortality because they too, though to a lesser degree than ventricular tachyarrhythmias, signify underlying electrical and/or structural abnormalities that negatively impact the prognosis of those patients who experience them compared to those who do not.

Another interesting hypothesis is that right ventricular pacing with a dual-chamber ICD may contribute to increased HF risk after ICD implant.[13] In the MADIT-II study, however, the risk of HF events was similar whether patients received a single- or dual-chamber ICD despite differences in right ventricular pacing (92% of patients with single-lead ICDs had no pacing, whereas 66% of patients with dual-chamber ICDs had cumulative RV pacing exceeding 50%).[3] Even if right ventricular pacing has a certain contribution to the adverse outcomes, the increased risk of HF after ICD implantation cannot be solely due to right ventricular pacing.[3]

These findings suggest that, in HF patients, an ICD shock is associated with a 2-to 5-fold increase in mortality, most commonly due to progressive HF.[1] It is not known whether the arrhythmia leading to ICD shock is a marker for worsening HF or whether the shock itself leads to worsening HF. Regardless of the individual factors causing greater HF events in current ICD populations, there appear to be multiple triggers that, when combined with high-risk patients, cause an increased HF risk. Heart failure patients with high-risk features such as NYHA functional class III, atrial fibrillation (AF), and ischemic cardiomyopathy require closer observation and management after ICD shock as sudden death risk is now transformed to an increased HF event risk.[3]

It is unknown whether the increase in risk in association to the appropriate ICD shocks is due to the ventricular arrhythmia (VA) or shocks and whether anti-tachycardia pacing

(ATP) termination can reduce this risk. To determine whether mortality in ICD patients is influenced by the type of therapy (shocks or ATP) delivered, Sweeney et al. evaluated the effects of baseline characteristics, VT, fast VT (FVT, 188–250 bpm), VF, and therapy type (shocks or ATP) on mortality among 2135 patients in four trials of ATP to reduce shocks.[14] The results revealed that patients with VA episodes and shocks have higher mortality (20% increased risk per shocked episode) than patients with neither or patients with VA treated only with ATP. In addition patients with more VA episodes and more shocks have higher mortality than patients with less of both. Interestingly, in this study, inappropriate shocked episodes were not associated with increased mortality risk. There are three potential explanations for these findings: (a) electrical trauma from shocks, but not ATP, increases risk; (b) VA episodes increase mortality risk irrespective of terminating therapy; (c) VA episodes and the shocks, but not ATP, increase mortality risk.[14] Interactions between adverse shock effects are possible for scenarios (a) and (c) such that patients with more VA episodes may be more susceptible to harm from shocks. When electrical therapy type was included in the statistical analysis, ATP-terminated VT and shocked VF remained significant predictors of death. However, the risk in either case was indistinguishable from the risk unqualified for therapy (4% for VT vs. 3% for VT ATP; 15% for VF vs. 16% for VF shocks) and uncoupling the mortality effect of therapy type from episode type was impossible. Therefore, it was not possible to conclude that shocks for VT are harmful and that ATP is harmless or that shocks for VF increase episode risk.[14] However, since 1/3 of FVT episodes were shocked and 2/3 ATP terminated, episode and therapy type mortality effects could be statistically uncoupled. FVT treated with ATP only was not associated with increased risk of death, whereas similar FVT episodes that were shocked increased the risk of death by 32% suggesting that shocks are associated with increased risk and ATP is not.[14] The majority of shocks (60%) were for FVT, and 72% of shocked patients had at least one shock for FVT, making shocked FVT the most prevalent type of shocked episode and the dominant shock effect in the mortality models. Most shocks that were delivered in this study were for FVT and occurred at a 12 times higher rate among patients who died, whereas shocks for VF occurred at a 8 times higher rate.

Time spent in VA was 7 times higher per month among patients who died, and episode durations were higher for all episode/therapy combinations and greatest for shocked episodes preceded by failed ATP (22-fold increase). In addition to receiving more shocks, patients who died had longer duration shocked episodes (including failed ATP) and spent more time in shocked episodes compared with survivors. It is possible that longer episode durations after failed ATP magnify the adverse effect of shocks.[14]

In summary, the results from the study of Sweeney et al. confirm that shocks are associated with increased risk of adverse outcomes while ATP is not. This is consistent with data from MADIT II where ATP, unlike shocks, was not associated with increased risk of death.[16]

3.2 Possible mechanisms for increased risk of negative outcomes associated with appropriate ICD shocks

The idea that shocks are associated with risk of death and HF in ICD patients is not new. A commonly held interpretation is that VA is a marker for clinical deterioration, shocks are harmless, and the increased risk reflects progression of the myocardial disease.[1, 14, 17]

An alternative explanation is that shocks may causally increase risks of HF and death. In MADIT II, the risk of first and recurrent HF hospitalization increased by 90% and 74%, respectively, after appropriate shocks.[10] Survival after the first appropriate shock was 80% at

1 year. This was significantly less than the survival before the first shock, and the nonsudden cardiac death rate increased 17%.[8]

Shock-related myocardial injury has been investigated extensively. Large shock field strengths destroy cardiac myocytes causing biomarker release, which increases with shock strength and proximity to recent MI.[11, 12, 18] The severity of post-resuscitation myocardial depression increases with shock strength, and is inversely related to survival.[19] Repetitive shocks may cause cardiovascular collapse and death due to electromechanical dissociation.[14]

One reasonable hypothesis would be that the specific type of the arrhythmia episode may precondition the myocardium to the adverse effects of shocks and that factors unique to spontaneous ventricular arrhythmias magnify these effects, particularly in ATP-unresponsive ventricular episodes.

Investigations of shock-related myocardial injury have focused on acute effects that may be insufficient to account for reduced survival after appropriate shocks.[14] Other mechanisms may be important. Shocks may activate signaling pathways in the molecular cascade of HF. The clinical consequence may manifest months after shocks.

In contrast to the data on ICD shocks, there is no evidence that ATP has adverse cardiac effects. ATP termination of VT or FVT, unlike shocks, does not cause biomarker release [20] or reduce ventricular pump function.[21]

3.3 Clinical implications

Twenty-two percent to 35% of patients will receive appropriate ICD therapy for VT or VF within 3 years of implant, with an annual ICD shock rate of 5%.[1, 3, 8] Despite the possible increase risk of death and HF with shocks, ICDs prolong survival.[14] Near total reliance on shocks may have underestimated the ICD survival benefit in the above-mentioned clinical trials. The SCD-HeFT study was designed to provide ICD therapy that consisted of shock-only, single lead therapy for rapid, sustained VT or VF. No dual chamber or ATP therapy was allowed.[3] The incidence of appropriate shock for VT or VF was 22.4%. Sixty-seven percent of patients received no ICD therapy. In the MADIT-II study, dual-chamber devices were used with the capability of ATP or shock therapy.

Since VF can only be terminated with shocks, uncoupling therapy from episode risk could be indirectly addressed with graded shock energies.[14] Strategies to minimize shocks by using ATP as first line device therapy when possible,[22] decrease shock energies, and reduce the burden of ventricular arrhythmias by using antiarrhythmic drugs and substrate modification may further improve survival in ICD patients.[14] There are several other strategies that were proven effective in reducing device shocks. In a recent study by Desai and colleagues In the present study of 549 patients with heart failure and ICDs, smoking significantly increased the incidence of appropriate ICD shocks 3.7 times, and the use of statins significantly reduced appropriate ICD shocks by 46%.[23] This is consistent with previous results from the MADIT II trial.[24, 25]

4. Inappropriate ICD shocks

Inappropriate ICD discharges result from the inability to distinguish supraventricular from ventricular arrhythmias, abnormal arrhythmia sensing or mechanical problems such as lead fracture, insulation break, and lead dislodgement. The shocks are painful, psychologically disturbing, potentially arhythmogenic and possibly associated with worse survival.

4.1 Incidence, mechanisms, and predictors of inappropriate shocks

An important contribution to the literature on the epidemiology of inappropriate ICD therapy was provided by the investigators of the MADIT II trial.[16] The authors reported an incidence of inappropriate shocks of 11.5 % with a cumulative 1 and 2 year event rate of 10% and 13% respectively.[16] In other studies such as AVID, PainFREE Rx, SCD-HeFT the incidence of inappropriate shocks was reported to be 20%, 15% and 32% respectively.[1, 26] The MIRACLE ICD study reported an incidence of inappropriate detection of 32% but not all detections resulted in an ICD discharge. Although the incidence of inappropriate ICD shocks was found to be somewhere between 10% and 35% in all the studies available in literature, the ratio of inappropriate ICD shocks over the appropriate shocks varies widely depending on the population that was studied. The highest ratio is expected to occur in patients who receive ICDs for primary prevention where the incidence of appropriate ICD shocks is relatively low. The majority of these patients experience the first inappropriate shock after a mean period of 17±15 months from the device implantation. The cumulative percent rate was found to be around 7% at 1 year, 13% at 3 years and 18% at 5 years. Approximately a third of the patients who receive one inappropriate shock typically receive the second one after a mean period of 11±11 months with the cumulative event rate of 28%, 49%, and 55% at 1 year, 3 years and 5 years respectively after the first shock.[27]

The most common causes of inappropriate ICD shocks are supraventricular tachycardia episodes and inappropriate sensing. Of all supraventricular tachycardias, AF with rapid ventricular response is the most common cause of an inappropriate ICD shock. This occurs because most ICDs are programmed to recognize VT when the heart rate exceeds a threshold value and SVTs may do so. Device companies have developed algorithms by which ICDs may differentiate VT from SVT using such parameters as sudden onset, rhythm stability and electrogram template matching. These strategies have demonstrated little impact in reducing discharges for SVT in part due to limited rhythm discrimination, because VT and SVT can mimic each other, and in greater part because they are probably little utilized by programming physicians.

Atrial fibrillation (AF) is a common finding in patients with low left ventricular ejection fraction and HF symptoms. Among HF patients, AF can occur with a prevalence of as high as 50% in patients with New York Heart Association (NYHA) functional class IV. Patients with HF and ICDs who also have AF have a significantly higher risk of experiencing inappropriate ICD shocks than patients without AF. Furthermore, patients with permanent AF seem to have doubled risk of developing an inappropriate shock, and patients with paroxysmal or persistent AF are exposed to a tripled risk of developing inappropriate ICD shocks when compared with the patients without any history of AF.

There are other risk factors for inappropriate shocks in addition to supraventricular tachyarrhythmias. Age younger than 70 years, nonischemic cardiomyopathy, non-use of statins, smoking, and interim appropriate ICD shocks were reported to be independent predictors of inappropriate ICD shocks.[16, 24, 29]

The MADIT II trial data analysis as well as other recent studies shows a significant 3-fold increase in the risk of inappropriate ICD shocks among current smokers. The overall risk of inappropriate ICD therapy was significantly increased among current smokers (20%) compared to past smokers (14%) and patients who never smoked (11%). This difference was mainly due to the increased numbers of ICD shocks in the current smokers group. The main causes of the ICD shocks in these groups were supraventricular tachycardia and sinus tachycardia, which were more frequent in current smokers than in past and never-smokers.

Tobacco smoke causes sympathetic stimulation as well as increased platelet reactivity and endothelial dysfunction, tachycardia and high blood pressure, all of these leading to supraventricular tachycardia which could potentially induce inappropriate ICD shocks.[1, 24]
In some cases the treatment for ventricular arrhythmias can precipitate AF and initiate an inappropriate ICD discharge. An inappropriate therapy itself causing VT can lead to an appropriate ICD discharge as well. Most of the patients who received an ICD for VT or VF have predisposing factors that are common for VT and AF, which also makes them more prone in developing AF and increases their risk of inappropriate discharge. [30, 31]
Recent studies have demonstrated that patients younger than seventy years old are at increased risk for experiencing inappropriate ICD shocks[24] due chiefly to sinus tachycardia episodes.[27]
One study has demonstrated that the cause of inappropriate shocks is partly dependent on the number of ICD leads. Patients with single chamber devices received more shocks for sinus tachycardia compared to those with dual chamber units (28% vs 8%) ,whereas patients with CRT devices received more shocks due to abnormal sensing compared to patients with single chamber ICDs (15% vs. 8 %).[27]

4.2 Prognostic importance of inappropriate ICD shocks

Data from ICD trials have demonstrated that inapropriate ICD discharges may compund the prognostic risk of appropriate shocks. Poole et al. found that among patients who received ICDs for primary prevention of SCD the risk of death doubled when inappropriate shocks were delivered in comparison to patients who did not receive shocks at all.[1] A patient who received an appropriate shock and an inappropriate shock has a risk of death increased by a factor of 11 when compared with a patient who received no shock at all. The patients who received at least two previous appropriate shocks and have received an inappropriate shock have a risk of death increased by 15 and additional inappropriate shocks do not result in further increase in the risk of death. Similar findings were reported in the MADIT II trial. Although previous studies reported appropriate shocks to be predictors of future CHF hospitalizations, in the MADIT II trial the inappropriate shocks did not predict future hospitalizations.[16]
It is uncertain why an inappropriate shock is associated with an increase in mortality. One possible explanation could be the fact that the development of AF, the most common cause of an inappropriate shock, in a patient with heart failure carries a worse prognosis.[32] Benjamin et al. showed that the occurrence of AF was associated with a 1.5 to 1.9-fold risk of all-cause mortality.[32] These findings were confirmed also in an ICD population by Borleffs and colleagues who found a 1.7 times increased risk of mortality in patients with permanent AF when compared with non-AF population. The highest mortality is shown by the patients who have permanent atrial fibrillation followed by those with persistent atrial fibrillation and then by patients with paroxysmal atrial fibrillation. [28]
Other causes that could explain the increase in mortality could be explained by the direct effect of the shocks on the myocardium. The presence of positive cardiac markers after inappropriate discharge suggests that the shock causes myocardial damage leading to ventricular dysfunction.[28, 33] Shocks with higher energy delivered are more likely to cause more myocardial damage. Tokano and colleagues demonstrated that shocks with energy greater than 9 J cause a 10% to 15% transient reduction of the cardiac index. The duration and the extent of the effect are proportional to the shock strength. The detrimental

homodynamic effect of a ventricular defibrillator shock appears to be due to the shock itself, and not to ventricular fibrillation. The latest conclusion was drawn from the observation that a similar degree of ventricular stunning was noted after shocks delivered during the baseline rhythm as with shocks that terminated ventricular fibrillation.[34]

4.3 Impact on psychology and life style

Delivery of an ICD shock, is often associated with increased psychological distress in patients and their families.[35, 36] The AVID trial extended these findings by demonstrating that patients who received more than one ICD shock within the initial year of implantation reported significant declines in physical functioning and mental well being.[37] Increased sadness, anxiety, fatigue, and nervousness were also found to be associated with more ICD discharges[38] Other studies reported that overall psychological distress was significantly correlated with the total number of ICD shocks a patient receives.[39]

4.4 Clinical implications

Ever since ICD therapy was developed technology improved constantly including the ability to differentiate supraventricular from ventricular tachyarrhythmias and to prevent inappropriate discharges. In spite of all the progress been made, recent research that assessed the incidence of inappropriate shocks in the ICDs implanted recently in comparison to those implanted a while ago did not show any improvement even more than that it appeared that the patients who received the ICDs more recently are exposed to a greater risk of developing an inappropriate shock. This phenomenon is mostly explained by the fact that guidelines for ICD implantation keep changing, shifting more towards primary prevention. The primary prevention group is represented by patients who usually have a more advanced underlying cardiac disease, which exposes them to a higher risk of developing AF, which is the number one cause of inappropriate discharge.[33] Criteria incorporated in the modern ICD algorithms used to discriminate ventricular from supraventricular tachycardia include rapidity of onset of the arrhythmia and QRS morphology.[40] Discriminating algorithms typically increase the specificity but at the same time they decrease the sensitivity for VT recognition.[41]

Despite widespread use of antiarrhythmic medications in patients with ICDs there are only a few studies documenting the efficacy of these therapies in this patient population. Sotalol and dofetilide when used as antiarrhythmic agents in patients with ICDs were found to reduce the risk of inappropriate shocks.[42, 43] Amiodarone was also found to be effective in preventing inappropriate shocks in patients with ICDs but it has a significant number of side effects and can lead to elevation of the defibrillation threshold (DFT).

In addition, the β-adrenergic blocking agents are efficacious antiarrhythmic drug therapies and can be effective in reducing the incidence of both supraventricular and ventricular arrhythmias in ICD patients.

Finally, trying to address other identifiable predictors of innapropiate shocks might be beneficial in terms of reducing both appropriate and inappropriate shocks: smoking cessation, treating illnesses that can cause sinus tachycardia, starting the patient on a statin if appropriate.

5. References

[1] Poole JE, Johnson GW, Hellkamp AS, Anderson J, Callans DJ, Raitt MH, Reddy RK, Marchlinski FE, Yee R, Guarnieri T, Talajic M, Wilber DJ, Fishbein DP, Packer DL,

Mark DB, Lee KL, Bardy GH. Prognostic importance of defibrillator shocks in patients with heart failure. *N Engl J Med.* 2008;359(10):1009-1017.

[2] A comparison of antiarrhythmic-drug therapy with implantable defibrillators in patients resuscitated from near-fatal ventricular arrhythmias. The Antiarrhythmics versus Implantable Defibrillators (AVID) Investigators. *N Engl J Med.* 1997;337(22):1576-1583.

[3] Mishkin JD, Saxonhouse SJ, Woo GW, Burkart TA, Miles WM, Conti JB, Schofield RS, Sears SF, Aranda JM, Jr. Appropriate evaluation and treatment of heart failure patients after implantable cardioverter-defibrillator discharge: time to go beyond the initial shock. *J Am Coll Cardiol.* 2009;54(22):1993-2000.

[4] Gehi AK, Mehta D, Gomes JA. Evaluation and management of patients after implantable cardioverter-defibrillator shock. *JAMA.* 2006;296(23):2839-2847.

[5] Moss AJ, Zareba W, Hall WJ, Klein H, Wilber DJ, Cannom DS, Daubert JP, Higgins SL, Brown MW, Andrews ML. Prophylactic implantation of a defibrillator in patients with myocardial infarction and reduced ejection fraction. *N Engl J Med.* 2002;346(12):877-883.

[6] Bardy GH, Lee KL, Mark DB, Poole JE, Packer DL, Boineau R, Domanski M, Troutman C, Anderson J, Johnson G, McNulty SE, Clapp-Channing N, Davidson-Ray LD, Fraulo ES, Fishbein DP, Luceri RM, Ip JH. Amiodarone or an implantable cardioverter-defibrillator for congestive heart failure. *N Engl J Med.* 2005;352(3):225-237.

[7] Epstein AE, DiMarco JP, Ellenbogen KA, Estes NA, 3rd, Freedman RA, Gettes LS, Gillinov AM, Gregoratos G, Hammill SC, Hayes DL, Hlatky MA, Newby LK, Page RL, Schoenfeld MH, Silka MJ, Stevenson LW, Sweeney MO, Smith SC, Jr., Jacobs AK, Adams CD, Anderson JL, Buller CE, Creager MA, Ettinger SM, Faxon DP, Halperin JL, Hiratzka LF, Hunt SA, Krumholz HM, Kushner FG, Lytle BW, Nishimura RA, Ornato JP, Riegel B, Tarkington LG, Yancy CW. ACC/AHA/HRS 2008 Guidelines for Device-Based Therapy of Cardiac Rhythm Abnormalities: a report of the American College of Cardiology/American Heart Association Task Force on Practice Guidelines (Writing Committee to Revise the ACC/AHA/NASPE 2002 Guideline Update for Implantation of Cardiac Pacemakers and Antiarrhythmia Devices) developed in collaboration with the American Association for Thoracic Surgery and Society of Thoracic Surgeons. *J Am Coll Cardiol.* 2008;51(21):e1-62.

[8] Moss AJ, Greenberg H, Case RB, Zareba W, Hall WJ, Brown MW, Daubert JP, McNitt S, Andrews ML, Elkin AD. Long-term clinical course of patients after termination of ventricular tachyarrhythmia by an implanted defibrillator. *Circulation.* 2004;110(25):3760-3765.

[9] Moss AJ, Hall WJ, Cannom DS, Daubert JP, Higgins SL, Klein H, Levine JH, Saksena S, Waldo AL, Wilber D, Brown MW, Heo M. Improved survival with an implanted defibrillator in patients with coronary disease at high risk for ventricular arrhythmia. Multicenter Automatic Defibrillator Implantation Trial Investigators. *N Engl J Med.* 1996;335(26):1933-1940.

[10] Goldenberg I, Moss AJ, Hall WJ, McNitt S, Zareba W, Andrews ML, Cannom DS. Causes and consequences of heart failure after prophylactic implantation of a defibrillator in the multicenter automatic defibrillator implantation trial II. *Circulation.* 2006;113(24):2810-2817.

[11] Blendea D, Blendea M, Banker J, McPherson CA. Troponin T elevation after implanted defibrillator discharge predicts survival. *Heart.* 2009;95(14):1153-1158.

[12] Hurst TM, Hinrichs M, Breidenbach C, Katz N, Waldecker B. Detection of myocardial injury during transvenous implantation of automatic cardioverter-defibrillators. *J Am Coll Cardiol.* 1999;34(2):402-408.

[13] Wilkoff BL, Cook JR, Epstein AE, Greene HL, Hallstrom AP, Hsia H, Kutalek SP, Sharma A. Dual-chamber pacing or ventricular backup pacing in patients with an implantable defibrillator: the Dual Chamber and VVI Implantable Defibrillator (DAVID) Trial. *JAMA.* 2002;288(24):3115-3123.

[14] Sweeney MO, Sherfesee L, DeGroot PJ, Wathen MS, Wilkoff BL. Differences in effects of electrical therapy type for ventricular arrhythmias on mortality in implantable cardioverter-defibrillator patients. *Heart Rhythm.*7(3):353-360.

[15] Tang W, Weil MH, Sun S, Yamaguchi H, Povoas HP, Pernat AM, Bisera J. The effects of biphasic and conventional monophasic defibrillation on postresuscitation myocardial function. *J Am Coll Cardiol.* 1999;34(3):815-822.

[16] Daubert JP, Zareba W, Cannom DS, McNitt S, Rosero SZ, Wang P, Schuger C, Steinberg JS, Higgins SL, Wilber DJ, Klein H, Andrews ML, Hall WJ, Moss AJ. Inappropriate implantable cardioverter-defibrillator shocks in MADIT II: frequency, mechanisms, predictors, and survival impact. *J Am Coll Cardiol.* 2008;51(14):1357-1365.

[17] Pacifico A, Ferlic LL, Cedillo-Salazar FR, Nasir N, Jr., Doyle TK, Henry PD. Shocks as predictors of survival in patients with implantable cardioverter-defibrillators. *J Am Coll Cardiol.* 1999;34(1):204-210.

[18] Nikolski VP, Efimov IR. Electroporation of the heart. *Europace.* 2005;7 Suppl 2:146-154.

[19] Xie J, Weil MH, Sun S, Tang W, Sato Y, Jin X, Bisera J. High-energy defibrillation increases the severity of postresuscitation myocardial dysfunction. *Circulation.* 1997;96(2):683-688.

[20] Runsio M, Kallner A, Kallner G, Rosenqvist M, Bergfeldt L. Myocardial injury after electrical therapy for cardiac arrhythmias assessed by troponin-T release. *Am J Cardiol.* 1997;79(9):1241-1245.

[21] Stoddard MF, Labovitz AJ, Stevens LL, Buckingham TA, Redd RR, Kennedy HL. Effects of electrophysiologic studies resulting in electrical countershock or burst pacing on left ventricular systolic and diastolic function. *Am Heart J.* 1988;116(2 Pt 1):364-370.

[22] Wathen MS, DeGroot PJ, Sweeney MO, Stark AJ, Otterness MF, Adkisson WO, Canby RC, Khalighi K, Machado C, Rubenstein DS, Volosin KJ. Prospective randomized multicenter trial of empirical antitachycardia pacing versus shocks for spontaneous rapid ventricular tachycardia in patients with implantable cardioverter-defibrillators: Pacing Fast Ventricular Tachycardia Reduces Shock Therapies (PainFREE Rx II) trial results. *Circulation.* 2004;110(17):2591-2596.

[23] Desai H, Aronow WS, Ahn C, Gandhi K, Hussain S, Lai HM, Sharma M, Frishman WH, Cohen M, Sorbera C. Risk factors for appropriate cardioverter-defibrillator shocks, inappropriate cardioverter-defibrillator shocks, and time to mortality in 549 patients with heart failure. *Am J Cardiol.*105(9):1336-1338.

[24] Goldenberg I, Moss AJ, McNitt S, Zareba W, Daubert JP, Hall WJ, Andrews ML. Cigarette smoking and the risk of supraventricular and ventricular tachyarrhythmias in high-risk cardiac patients with implantable cardioverter defibrillators. *J Cardiovasc Electrophysiol.* 2006;17(9):931-936.

[25] Vyas AK, Guo H, Moss AJ, Olshansky B, McNitt SA, Hall WJ, Zareba W, Steinberg JS, Fischer A, Ruskin J, Andrews ML. Reduction in ventricular tachyarrhythmias with statins in the Multicenter Automatic Defibrillator Implantation Trial (MADIT)-II. *J Am Coll Cardiol.* 2006;47(4):769-773.

[26] Anderson JL, Hallstrom AP, Epstein AE, Pinski SL, Rosenberg Y, Nora MO, Chilson D, Cannom DS, Moore R. Design and results of the antiarrhythmics vs implantable defibrillators (AVID) registry. The AVID Investigators. *Circulation.* 1999;99(13):1692-1699.

[27] van Rees JB, Borleffs CJ, de Bie MK, Stijnen T, van Erven L, Bax JJ, Schalij MJ. Inappropriate implantable cardioverter-defibrillator shocks: incidence, predictors, and impact on mortality. *J Am Coll Cardiol.*57(5):556-562.

[28] Borleffs CJ, van Rees JB, van Welsenes GH, van der Velde ET, van Erven L, Bax JJ, Schalij MJ. Prognostic importance of atrial fibrillation in implantable cardioverter-defibrillator patients. *J Am Coll Cardiol.*55(9):879-885.

[29] Jodko L, Kornacewicz-Jach Z, Kazmierczak J, Rzeuski R, Zielonka J, Kaliszczak R, Safranow K. Inappropriate cardioverter-defibrillator discharge continues to be a major problem in clinical practice. *Cardiol J.* 2009;16(5):432-439.

[30] Johnson NJ, Marchlinski FE. Arrhythmias induced by device antitachycardia therapy due to diagnostic nonspecificity. *J Am Coll Cardiol.* 1991;18(5):1418-1425.

[31] Florin TJ, Weiss DN, Peters RW, Shorofsky SR, Gold MR. Induction of atrial fibrillation with low-energy defibrillator shocks in patients with implantable cardioverter defibrillators. *Am J Cardiol.* 1997;80(7):960-962.

[32] Benjamin EJ, Wolf PA, D'Agostino RB, Silbershatz H, Kannel WB, Levy D. Impact of atrial fibrillation on the risk of death: the Framingham Heart Study. *Circulation.* 1998;98(10):946-952.

[33] Schluter T, Baum H, Plewan A, Neumeier D. Effects of implantable cardioverter defibrillator implantation and shock application on biochemical markers of myocardial damage. *Clin Chem.* 2001;47(3):459-463.

[34] Tokano T, Bach D, Chang J, Davis J, Souza JJ, Zivin A, Knight BP, Goyal R, Man KC, Morady F, Strickberger SA. Effect of ventricular shock strength on cardiac hemodynamics. *J Cardiovasc Electrophysiol.* 1998;9(8):791-797.

[35] Dougherty CM. Psychological reactions and family adjustment in shock versus no shock groups after implantation of internal cardioverter defibrillator. *Heart Lung.* 1995;24(4):281-291.

[36] Dunbar S ZZ, Smith P. Quality of life outcomes for ventricular arrhythmia patients: The PRIDE Study. *Circulation.* 2001;104 (Suppl II):3618.

[37] Schron EB, Exner DV, Yao Q, Jenkins LS, Steinberg JS, Cook JR, Kutalek SP, Friedman PL, Bubien RS, Page RL, Powell J. Quality of life in the antiarrhythmics versus implantable defibrillators trial: impact of therapy and influence of adverse symptoms and defibrillator shocks. *Circulation.* 2002;105(5):589-594.

[38] Heller SS, Ormont MA, Lidagoster L, Sciacca RR, Steinberg S. Psychosocial outcome after ICD implantation: a current perspective. *Pacing Clin Electrophysiol.* 1998;21(6):1207-1215.

[39] Herbst JH, Goodman M, Feldstein S, Reilly JM. Health-related quality-of-life assessment of patients with life-threatening ventricular arrhythmias. *Pacing Clin Electrophysiol.* 1999;22(6 Pt 1):915-926.

[40] Higgins SL, Lee RS, Kramer RL. Stability: an ICD detection criterion for discriminating atrial fibrillation from ventricular tachycardia. *J Cardiovasc Electrophysiol.* 1995;6(12):1081-1088.

[41] Luceri RM. Initial clinical experience with a dual chamber rate responsive implantable cardioverter defibrillator. *Pacing Clin Electrophysiol.* 2000;23(11 Pt 2):1986-1988.

[42] Pacifico A, Hohnloser SH, Williams JH, Tao B, Saksena S, Henry PD, Prystowsky EN. Prevention of implantable-defibrillator shocks by treatment with sotalol. d,l-Sotalol Implantable Cardioverter-Defibrillator Study Group. *N Engl J Med.* 1999;340(24):1855-1862.

[43] O'Toole M ONG, Kluger J. Efficacy and safety of oral dofetilide in patients with an implantable defibrillator: A multicenter study. *Circulation.* 1999;100:I794.

[44] Healey J, Connoly S. Life and death after ICD implantation. N Engl J Med. 2008;359(10):1058-1059.

4

Ventricular Tachyarrhythmias in Implantable Cardioverter Defibrillator Recipients: Differences Between Ischemic and Dilated Cardiomyopathies

Aldo Casaleggio[1], Tiziana Guidotto[2], Vincenzo Malavasi[3] and Paolo Rossi[4]
[1]*National Research Council, Biophysics Institute, Genova,*
[2]*St. Jude Medical Italia, Clinical Department, Agrate Brianza, Milano,*
[3]*Modena Polyclinic Hospital, Cardiology Division, Modena,*
[4]*San Martino Hospital, Cardiology Division, Genova,*
Italy

1. Introduction

Progress in implantable cardioverter-defibrillator (ICD) technology has led to significant improvements in the management of malignant ventricular tachyarrhythmias (VT) from patients with different etiologies [Henkel & Witt 2006, Javaray & Monahan 2005]. Figure 1 depicts the case of a patient who experienced a malignant ventricular fibrillation rapidly resolved by the ICD.

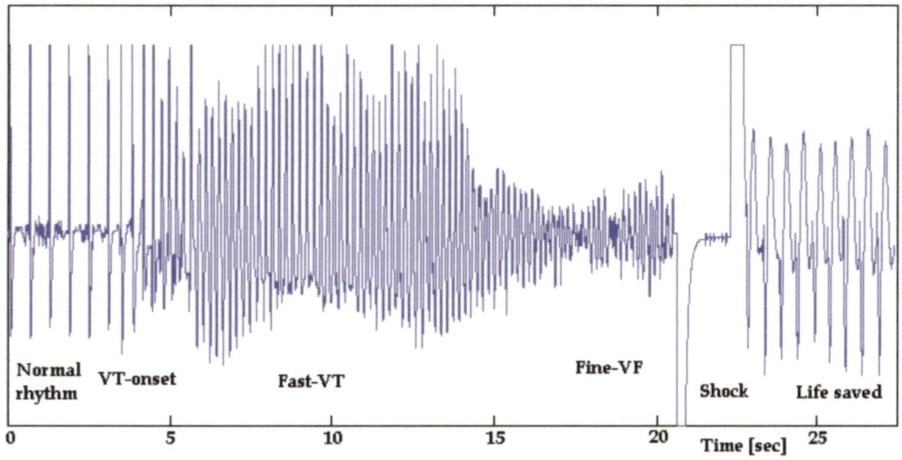

Fig. 1. Example of malignant ventricular tachycardia degenerating in ventricular fibrillation, automatically recognized and treated by the ICD.

In addition, the ability of these devices to record and store information on electrical cardiac activity immediately preceding the arrhythmia onset and during its course has enabled the assessment of the initiation pattern and characteristics of these arrhythmias. Eventually, at the end of the nineties, it has been shown that coronary artery disease (CAD) and dilated cardiomyopathy (DCM) underlie different mechanisms of spontaneous and induced VT [Pogwizd et al. 1998, Chung et al. 1997]; moreover ,differences in spontaneous VT from ICD recipients began to be investigated. Indeed, since the early 2000, various studies have analyzed intracardiac electrograms (EGMs) and initiation VT pattern [Gorenek et al. 2006, Taylor et al. 2000, Saeed et al. 2000], while others have investigated circadian distribution [Carson et al. 2000, Englund et al. 1999, Eksik et al. 2007, Taneda et al. 2001] of spontaneous VT in ICD patients. Some of these studies [Taylor et al. 2000, Saeed et al. 2000, Englund et al. 1999] have failed to detect differences in both the patterns of initiation and in EGMs between patients with different etiologies of heart disease. In contrast, differences in the circadian distribution were detected in other studies [Carson et al. 2000, Taneda et al. 2001], showing that patients with CAD had a peak of the VT episodes in the morning, whereas patients with non-ischemic cardiomyopathy and heart failure had a more uniform VT distribution during the light hours and a few episodes during the night. The main limitation of these studies lies in their definition of non-ischemic cardiomyopathy, which included different cardiac diseases such as dilated cardiomyopathy, hypertrophic cardiomyopathy, valvular heart disease, right ventricular dysplasia and others.

Unlike previous studies, this study focuses exclusively on patients with CAD and those with DCM. Therefore, by analyzing spontaneous VT from ICDs, we sought to determine whether there were differences in EGM characteristics obtained from far-field recordings, VT prevalence, initiation patterns and circadian distribution between patients with CAD and DCM. A subset of this study was preliminarily presented [Casaleggio et al. 2008].

2. Methods

2.1 Electa registry

Sixty-seven patients were enrolled in the ElectA Registry (Electrogram Analysis) which included subjects undergoing implantation of St. Jude Medical single chamber ICD devices (models: Contour, Profile and Angstrom) for secondary prevention of aborted sudden cardiac death (SCD) due to ventricular fibrillation or sustained VT episodes (with duration greater than 30 sec). Among them, 46 had ischemic cardiomyopathy due to CAD, 17 had primary DCM and 4 had other etiology: one Brugada Syndrome, one RV Dysplasia and two hypertrophic cardiomyopathies.

ICDs allowed acquisitions of the EGMs in bipolar or far-field modes. In bipolar mode, EGMs were recorded between distal coil and electrocatheter tip at the right ventricular lead tip, and filtered with an high pass at 12 Hz. In far-field mode, EGMs were recorded between the distal coil and the active can of the device without low frequency filtration. In our previous study [Casaleggio et al. 2006], we examined the differences between bipolar and far-field recordings, and observed that the two modes of acquisition should not be combined to avoid characterization errors. Furthermore, far-field recordings easily recognized pacing beats, allowed a better definition of the T-wave in sinus rhythm and a higher discrimination of the QRS morphology for the off-line diagnosis of VT (see Figure 2).

In order to study VT-onset, ICDs were programmed to store EGMs of 2 minutes at a sampling frequency of 250 Hz, that allowed up to three EGMs recordings on a single channel at each follow-up. Moreover, since storage was triggered on VT initiation (when VT is shorter than 2 minutes), the protocol required a pre-trigger of 20 sec. at minimum to

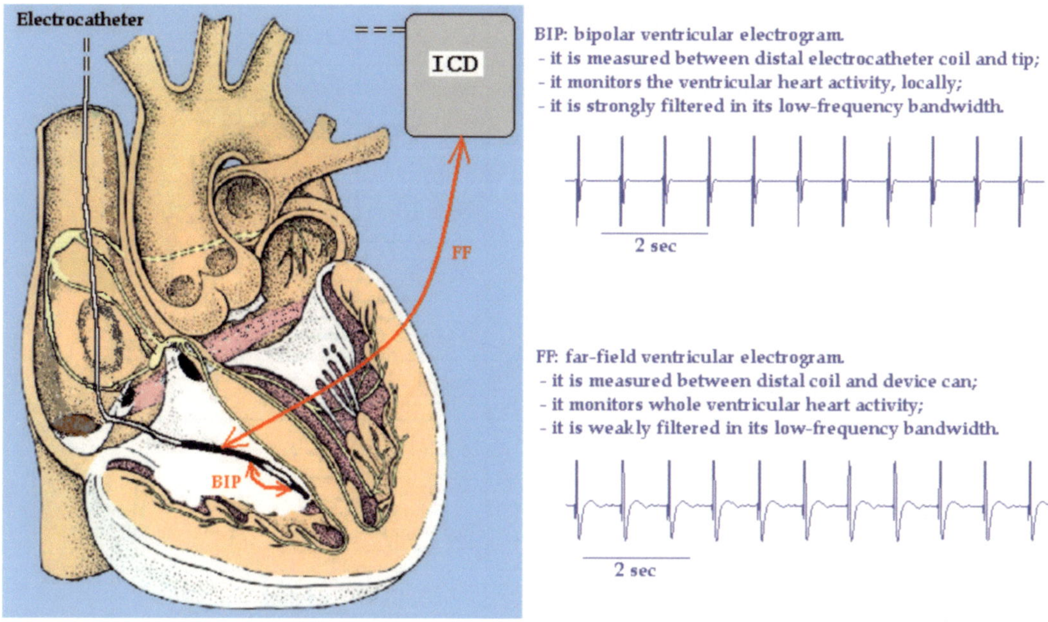

Fig. 2. Schematic of bipolar and far-field EGMs from ICDs. In the right side of the panel the main characteristics of the two types of recordings are described and examples are shown.

monitor basal rhythm immediately before VT initiation. Patients gave written consent for the implantation , follow-up and planned evaluations; they were identified by their ICD serial numbers. Patients were excluded from the ElectA study if they had an indication to dual-chamber ICD implantation, or refused to consent. ICD settings were at the discretion of the physician, except for a pre-trigger at 20 seconds. No requirements were proposed either for VT- therapy (rate cutoff and monitoring zone) or bradycardia pacing, although all clinicians programmed a lower rate in VVI mode at 50-60 beats per minute.
Clinical information for each patient including age, gender, heart disease, left ventricular ejection fraction, and antiarrhythmic drug therapy at the time of ICD implant, were documented by review of clinical records. Information on VT events and circadian distribution were retrieved from the log file of the ICD device. ICD follow-up was routinely performed every 3-4 months and whenever patients felt palpitations, dizziness or shock.

2.2 Patient population

The present study focused only on patients with CAD or DCM. The CAD group included 46 patients (26 of which had VT episodes) with a history of previous myocardial infarction, angina, coronary angioplasty or coronary by-pass surgery. The DCM group included 17 patients (11 of which had VT episodes) with progressive cardiac dilation and left ventricular systolic dysfunction (ejection fraction less than 0.40), without significant CAD defined as greater than 50% stenosis in at least one vessel by coronary angiography. In all patients secondary etiology was excluded by clinical evaluation of potential causes such as alcoholism, thyroid disease, viral infection of the heart, valvular heart abnormalities, heredofamilial disease, or toxic drugs. No endomyocardial biopsy was obtained.
The baseline characteristics of CAD and DCM patients that experienced spontaneous malignant VT episodes are reported in Table 1.

	CAD	DCM	p
N. of patients with VT	26	11	
Clinical Characteristics			
Age (years)	70 ± 10	64 ± 12	n.s. $^{(\alpha)}$
Gender (male/female)	23 / 3	10 / 1	n.s. $^{(\beta)}$
Follow-up (months)	33 ± 10	24 ± 13	<0.03 $^{(\alpha)}$
Ejection Fraction (%)	35 ± 8	31 ± 9	n.s. $^{(\alpha)}$
NYHA Class: I / II+III (n)	2 / 24	2 / 9	n.s. $^{(\beta)}$
Basal rhythm: Sinus / Atrial fibrillation (n)	23 / 3	8 / 3	n.s. $^{(\beta)}$
Treatment at ICD implant: Amiodarone , n (%) Beta-blockers , n (%) Amiodarone + Beta-blockers , n (%) None or other drugs , n (%)	 14 (54%) 1 (4%) 3 (11%) 8 (31%)	 3 (27%) 1 (9%) 1 (9%) 6 (55%)	

Table 1. Clinical Characteristics of CAD and DCM patients with VT episodes; $^{(\alpha)}$ Statistical analysis performed with Student T-test; $^{(\beta)}$ Statistical analysis performed by chi-square test.

2.3 Modes of VT initiation and evaluated EGM characteristics

All VT episodes (monomorphic and polymorphic VT and ventricular fibrillation) were analyzed by cardiologists. VT were identified by a sudden increase in heart rate (defined as a rhythm greater than 140 beats per minute) along with a change in EGM morphology from the baseline rhythm. Arrhythmias due to atrial fibrillation or atrial flutter were excluded from the analysis. Using EGMs, VT initiation was characterized as follows: VT initiated by a premature ventricular contraction (PVC), defined as PVC pattern (Fig. 3A); VT initiated by a short-long-short cycle (SLS pattern, Fig. 3B); VT initiated with a PVC immediately after a paced ventricular beat (PM pattern, Fig. 3C). The pause preceding paced beats was considered appropriate if it was consistent with the programmed pacing escape interval.

For each VT episode the following features were analyzed: (i) *VT-cycle* defined as the median value of the VT cycles, in milliseconds (msec); (ii) *Coupling interval* (CI) taken as the interval between the first beat of VT and the previous baseline beat, in msec; (iii) *Prematurity index* (PI) calculated by normalizing the coupling interval to the preceding RR interval; (iv) *Median heart cycle* of the 20 seconds immediately preceding VT onset (HC-PreVT), in msec; (v) number of PVC and (vi) number of paced beats in the 20 sec preceding VT. The morphological analysis of PVC and VT was not considered.

Circadian distribution analysis was made over a 3 hour time interval, performing a sufficiently detailed analysis and an adequate number of VT episodes in each time interval.

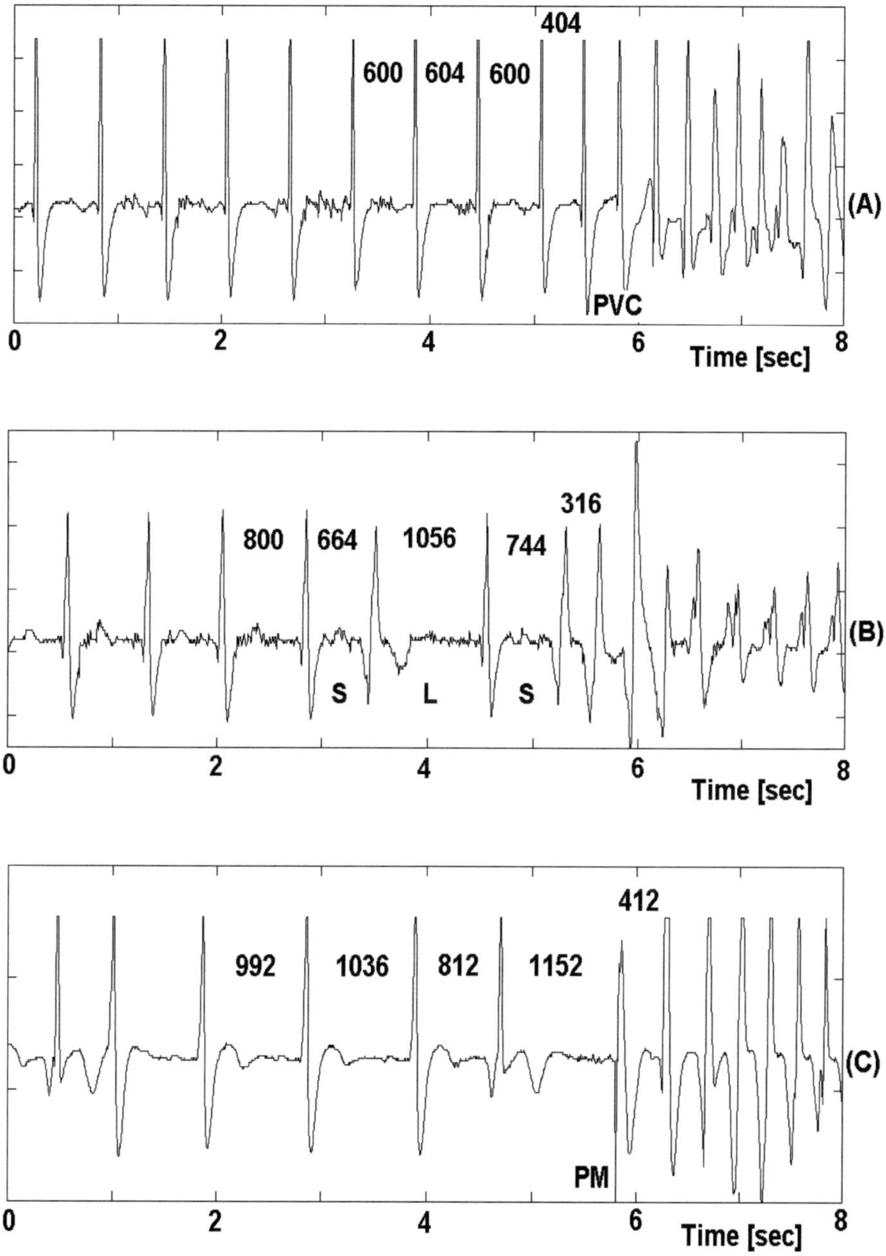

Fig. 3. Examples of tachyarrhythmia initiation patterns from ICD recordings: Panel (A) shows a PVC onset, Panel (B) is a short-long-short (SLS) onset, Panel (C) illustrates a tachyarrhythmia initiated immediately after a paced beat (PM onset); Numbers between R-peaks indicate RR intervals in msec.

2.4 Statistical analysis

Intervals and continuous variables are expressed as mean ± standard deviation. Differences between groups are analyzed using the Student T-test for continuous variables or the Chi-square test for categorical variables. Statistical significance is assumed when $p<0.05$. The number of VT per patient, and the number and type of VT-onset experienced by the patients, are considered together with their average values. Differences between average values are analyzed using the Student T-test.

Circadian distributions are modeled by polynomial (fifth order) and harmonic regression (two harmonics). It is expected that distributions with peaks and dumb-peaks can better be fitted by harmonic models, while smooth distributions would be better modeled as polynomials. Goodness of fit of the regression models has been tested using the coefficient of determination R^2, defined as in equation (1):

$$R^2(y) = 1 - \frac{\sum_i (y_i - \hat{y}_i)^2}{\sum_i (y_i - \overline{y})^2} \tag{1}$$

In equation (1) the value of y_i represents the measured variable for each 3-hour interval, $\overline{y}_i$ is its mean value, and $\hat{y}_i$ is the approximation obtained by the regression model. No formal sample size calculation has been performed.

3. Results

A total of 218 VT episodes were recorded in far-field mode during a follow up period of 30 ± 12 months. The analysis included all VT episodes requiring ICD therapy by antitachycardia pacing or shock cardioversion, as well as non-treated VT that recovered spontaneously. In particular 165 VT episodes which occurred in 37 patients, including 26 CAD patients (79 episodes) and 11 DCM patients (86 VT episodes) were analyzed. The remaining 53 VT episodes, (29 from DCM and 24 from CAD patients) could not be analyzed because, lasting more than 2 minutes, VT initiation was not available for ICD programmable setting. No under-sensing was observed.

As shown in Table 2, there were significant differences between CAD and DCM patients with VT episodes. In particular, DCM patients experienced a significantly higher number of VT episodes and more variable pattern of VT initiation.

Table 3 presents the statistical analysis of EGM features associated with specific VT initiation patterns in patients with CAD or DCM. There were no significant differences between CAD and DCM groups. However, within each group, the SLS and PM patterns showed a significantly lower prematurity index than the PVC pattern. In addition, the PM pattern demonstrated a significantly longer heart cycle preVT versus PVC and SLS ($p < 0.01$).

Figures 4 and 5 depict the circadian distributions of VT episodes in CAD and DCM patients, with an analysis in the overall groups (Fig. 4) and in subgroups with different patterns of VT initiation (Fig. 5). Figure 4 shows the presence of the two peaks in CAD patients, and a more uniformly distribution during daylight hours with a few VT episodes during the night in DCM patients.

	CAD	DCM	P
Number of patients with VT	26	11	
Analysis of the 20 sec basal rhythm preceding VT-onset			
Paced beats / All beats	1 / 28	1 / 27	n.s. $^{(\beta)}$
Premature ventricular contraction / All beats	2 / 27	3 /27	n.s. $^{(\beta)}$
Analysis of VT episodes			
Number of VT episodes	79	86	
Number of VT episodes per patient, mean ±SD	3 ± 2	8 ± 5	<0.02 $^{(\alpha)}$
Analysis of the VT-onset patterns			
Total number of VT per pattern:			
PVC, n (%)	59 (75%)	51 (59%)	n.s. $^{(\gamma)}$
SLS, n (%)	13 (16%)	22 (26%)	
PM, n (%)	7 (9%)	13 (15%)	
Number of patients with 1, 2 or 3 patterns:			
Patients with a single initiation pattern, n (%)	22 (85%)	5 (45%)	< 0.01 $^{(\delta)}$
Patients with two initiation patterns, n (%)	4 (15%)	3 (27.5%)	
Patients with three initiation patterns, n (%)	0 (0%)	3 (27.5%)	
Average number of patterns per patient, mean ±SD	1.1 ± 0.4	1.8± 0.9	< 0.01 $^{(\alpha)}$

Table 2. Analysis of VT episodes in patients with CAD or DCM; Different statistical tests were applied: $^{(\alpha)}$ Statistical analysis is performed with Student T-test; $^{(\beta)}$ Statistical analysis is performed by chi-square test; $^{(\gamma)}$ chi-square test is done on 3x2 table to test different *Number of VT per pattern* in CAD vs. DCM; $^{(\delta)}$ chi-square test is computed on 3x2 table to test different *Number of patients with 1, 2 or 3 patterns* in CAD vs. DCM patients.

	CAD Patients			DCM Patients		
VT onset	PVC	SLS	PM	PVC	SLS	PM
# of Episodes	59	13	7	51	22	13
VT cycle (msec)	356±62	325±45	298±68	323±48	343±44	332±85
CI (msec)	497±147	515±70	600±136	499±162	542±112	533±125
PI	0.75±0.18	0.56±0.11*	0.5±0.12*	0.76±0.22	0.62±0.12*	0.48±0.14*+
HC-PreVT (msec)	697±170	663±112	1018±121*+	665±142	716±146	923±151*+

Table 3. EGM features associated with specific VT onset patterns in patients with CAD or DCM. Statistical significance is indicated as follows: * p <0.01 versus PVC within the same etiology group; + p<0.01 versus SLS within the same etiology group. Legend: VT patterns are defined as follows: PVC: VT initiated by a premature ventricular contraction; SLS: VT initiated by a short-long-short cycle; PM: VT initiated with a PVC immediately after a paced beat. CAD: coronary artery disease; DCM: dilated cardiomyopathy; CI: coupling interval, PI: prematurity index, HC-PreVT: heart cycle in the 20 seconds preceding VT-onset.

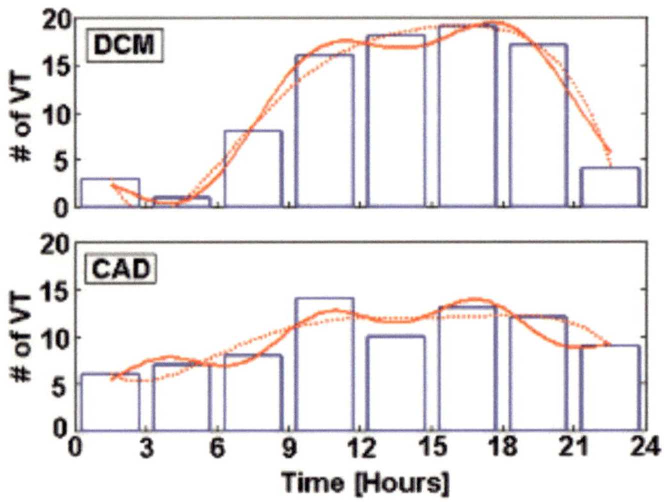

Fig. 4. Circadian distribution over a 3 hour time interval of CAD and DCM patients along with polynomial (dashed line) and harmonic (solid line) regression models.

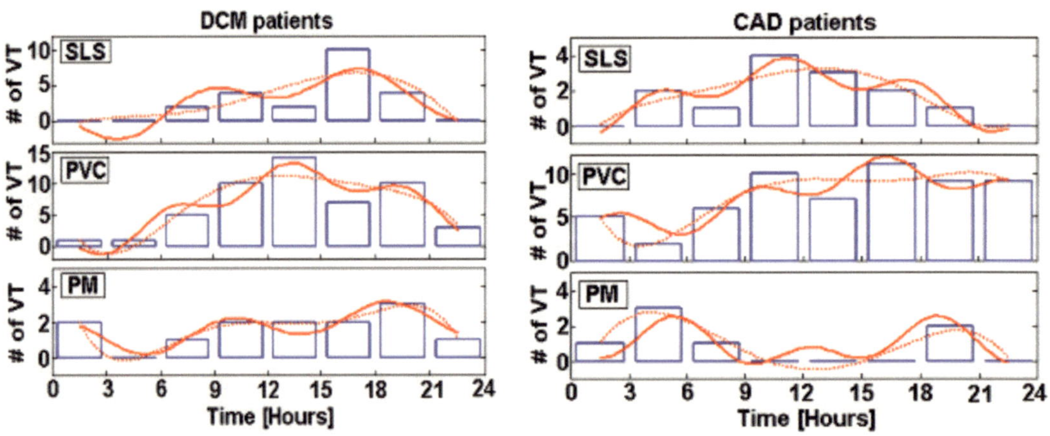

Fig. 5. Circadian distribution over a 3 hour time interval of CAD and DCM patients separated for the three different modes of onset. Corresponding polynomial (dashed line) and harmonic (solid line) regression models are shown.

To substantiate the observation that CAD and DCM population have different circadian distribution of VT episodes, the coefficients of determination (R^2), corresponding to the harmonic and polynomial regression models depicted in Figure 4, are computed. VT circadian distribution of CAD patients is better approximated by a harmonic model (R^2=0.963 vs. R^2=0.767 of polynomial regression). In DCM patients, harmonic and polynomial regression lead to similar R^2 values (R^2=0.983 vs. R^2=0.997, respectively), although the higher R^2 value is obtained approximating circadian distribution using a polynomial model.

Finally, determination coefficients of circadian distributions computed for homogeneous VT initiation pattern (PVC, SLS and PM) are resumed in Table 4.

	CAD Patients			DCM Patients		
	PVC	SLS	PM	PVC	SLS	PM
Harmonic model	**0.84**	**0.92**	0.71	0.78	**0.91**	0.85
Polynomial model	0.83	0.77	**0.9**	**0.86**	0.68	**0.98**

Table 4. Determination coefficient for harmonic and polynomial regressions: differences between CAD and DCM patients with similar VT-initiation patterns. Better performances are indicated in bold.

4. Discussion

The aim of this study was to determine whether there were differences in spontaneous VT initiation patterns and circadian distribution between ICD patients with CAD and DCM. Analysis of VT onset identified episodes triggered by a premature beat and two patterns of VT preceded by short-long-short cycles. The latter includes the SLS onset, which can be viewed as a spontaneous form, and the PM onset in which the ICD device facilitates VT initiation during anti-bradycardia pacing.

Significant differences between CAD and DCM were observed in the number of VT per patient and in the variability of the VT onset pattern (see Table 2). Patients with DCM had a significantly higher number of VT episodes despite clinical characteristics, ejection fraction and NYHA class were similar to CAD patients. It should be noted, as reported in Table 1, that the duration of follow-up was significantly longer in the CAD group, making the observation of a lower number of VT episodes in this group even more significant.

Other EGM features such as VT-rate, coupling interval and prematurity index, as well as those obtained from the EGM in the 20 sec preceding VT-onset (heart cycle, average number of PVC and of paced beats) were also studied (see Table 2 and 3) and, consistent with previous observations, no significant differences between CAD and DCM groups were observed. This might indicate that the studied EGM parameters do not express the intrinsic differences in the cardiac substrate of the two etiologies, as they are shown in the literature [Pogwizd et al. 1998, Sarter et al. 1998].

4.1 VT initiation patterns

In the literature the PVC onset is the most frequent mode of VT initiation [Taylor et al. 2000, Saeed et al. 2000]; SLS onset has been described as an arrhythmogenic mechanism [El-Sherif et al. 1999] distinct from PVC onset also in ICD recipients [Sarter et al. 1998]. Finally PM onset, observed only in case studies at the end of the nineties [Vlay & Vlay 1997], has been observed recently to occur in 8% - 15% of VT episodes in ICD patients [Sweeney et al. 2007].

Premature ventricular contraction (PVC) was the most frequent VT initiation pattern, especially in CAD patients.

Our results are consistent with findings from other authors [Gorenek et al. 2006, Taylor et al. 2000, Saeed et al. 2000], who underscored the importance of the initiation pattern of sustained VT in patients with ICDs. Gorenek et al. [Gorenek et al. 2006] and Saeed et al. [Saeed et al. 2000] analyzed the differences between VT onset preceded by several immediate PVCs (denominated extrasystolic onset) and VT with sudden onset, showing that extrasystolic onset was the most common pattern of VT initiation and was associated with lower ejection fraction. Sudden-onset initiation was more common with better preserved systolic function. Non sudden onset episodes required higher levels of shock energy and more frequent multiple shock achievements than sudden onset episodes [Gorenek et al. 2006].

In the present study the analysis of the modes of VT-onset indicated that 12% of VT initiate immediately after a paced beat, which may suggest a proarrhythmic effect of pacing in some patients [Sweeney et al. 2007, Himmrich et al. 2003]. These results are consistent with recent findings: Sweeney et al [Sweeney et al. 2007] found a 9.4% rate of VT initiated immediately after anti-bradycardia pacing in patients with a single chamber ICD, such as those used in our study. In our study the prevalence of VT with PM-onset was higher in DCM (15%) than CAD (9%), but statistical analysis with chi-square test shows that this difference is not significant ($p<0.28$). On the contrary, a statistically significant difference between CAD and DCM populations is obtained from the analysis of the number of initiation pattern indicating a more heterogeneous VT-onset in DCM patients (see Table 2). In particular, in 3 DCM patients all the three initiation patterns are present, while most of CAD initiated their VT always with the same mode.

Results in Table 3 indicate EGM features do not allow discriminating differences between CAD and DCM, suggesting that EGM features do not correlate with the cardiac disease substrate. However, in each group, significantly higher prematurity index and median heart cycle PreVT were observed in VT with PM-onset with respect to other VT initiation modes. The HC_PreVT can be explained by observing that anti-bradycardia pacing is a consequence of a low spontaneous heart rate. The significantly higher PI of PM-onset episodes, observed both in CAD and DCM patients, deserves further investigation.

4.2 Circadian distribution

In the literature the circadian distributions of VT episodes in the CAD population has been studied and a non-uniform distribution with clear peaks in the morning and afternoon has been observed [Englund et al. 1999, Eksik et al. 2007]. Results are controversial in the case of non-ischemic patients. While in some papers [Englund et al. 1999, Anand et al. 2007] non-ischemic disease presents circadian distribution similar to ischemic patients, in other studies [Carson et al. 2000, Taneda et al. 2001] non-ischemic patients do not have the morning peak and circadian distribution is almost uniformly distributed during daylight hours. The present study shows the presence of the two peaks in CAD patients, and a more uniformly distribution during daylight hours in DCM patients (see Fig. 4). This conclusion is further supported by our observation that the timing of VT-onset in CAD and DCM populations are described by structurally different statistical models, with harmonic and polynomial regression providing the best fitting function in CAD and DCM, respectively. The finding that the circadian distribution of VT in CAD patients is better described by a harmonic function (such as a bimodal activity) may suggest that the underlying arrhythmogenic mechanism could be oscillating during the 24-hour period, as is the case of the autonomic sympathetic-vagal balance. This hypothesis is supported by Taneda et al. who described a much higher peak of VT in the morning in patients not taking beta-blockers vs. patients who did [Figure 2 in Taneda et al. 2001]. Similarly, Dorian suggested that sympathetic activation can lead to a distributed shortening or, in some cases, prolonged action potential in the substrate, increasing the risk for reentrant arrhythmia [Dorian 2005].

By contrast, the result that the DCM circadian distribution is polynomial rather than harmonic, may suggest a different underlying mechanism at the basis of VT initiation. The observation that almost all VT occur during the day-light and almost none during the night, might lead to the hypothesis that sympathetic tone could be involved. In fact, Pogwizd described that a cardiac preserved beta-receptor responsiveness might likely facilitate early and delayed after-depolarizations, and, consequently, a triggered activity [Pogwizd et al. 2001, Pogwizd et al. 2004].

Such considerations might lead to speculate that sympatho-vagal tone changings could facilitate a reentry in the CAD group, while a higher sympathetic tone could determine a dangerous triggered activity in the DCM one.

It is noteworthy that the three different initiation patterns of VT episodes also show differences in the circadian distribution. (Figure 5 and Table 4).

VT initiated with PM pattern are better described, in both DCM and CAD patients, by a polynomial model. Distribution is almost uniform during the observed 24 hours in the DCM group , while it is mostly focused during the night in the CAD group. Although the number of VT is small (7 PM-onset in CAD and 13 in DCM), the result in the CAD population may be consistent with a lower heart rate occurring during the night, promoting a greater anti-bradycardia pacing intervention . It is less obvious to explain the finding in DCM, because the PM-onset occurs almost uniformly during the whole day. An increased prevalence of post-extrasystolic pauses distributed during the whole day, determining a frequent pacing escape, is more likely.

Circadian distribution of SLS patterns are well described by a harmonic models in both CAD (R^2 = 0.92 vs 0.77 for polynomial model) and DCM (R^2 = 0.91 vs 0.68 for polynomial model) with VT initiation especially between 9 a.m. to 6 p.m. in CAD, while it is evident a very strong peak between 3 p.m. to 6 p.m. in DCM patients.

Finally, the distribution of the PVC patterns is better described by a polynomial regression in the DCM group (R^2=0.86 vs. 0.78 for harmonic regression) with a peak in the middle of the day and no VT during the night (hour range: 0-6 a.m.); a different behavior is observed in the CAD group where a harmonic model fits slightly better (R^2=0.84 vs. 0.83 for polynomial model), with distribution showing small peaks between 9 a.m. and 12 a.m. and 3 p.m. to 6 p.m.

4.3 Limitations

The main limitations of this registry lie in the small number of patients and in the lack of endomyocardial biopsy in the DCM group. In addition, only single chamber ICDs were considered: they may present increased risk of PM-onset vs dual and three-chamber ICDs [Sweeney et al. 2007]. About the pharmacological treatment, the only detailed information was referred to implant date: eventual changes, during the follow-up period, were not collected.

Moreover, to examine the basal heart rhythm before the VT initiation, a good quality EGM at 250 Hz was obtained. As a consequence, for technical reasons, the ICD diagnostic parameters were programmed to store at the most three VT episodes. This setting, however, could have caused a lack of some episodes. For instance, in a DCM patient with some VT storms, successfully treated with the anti-tachycardia pacing, it was not possible to analyze all the episodes, but only the latest ones. In order to limit these drawbacks, the same settings were used for CAD and DCM groups and the follow-up was performed periodically, (minimum of 3 to maximum 6 months) unless the ICD delivered a shock. In that case, the patient was invited to contact the hospital for a visit as soon as possible and data were retrieved by the ICD. It is authors' opinion that the frequent follow-up could be sufficient to minimize the number of undetected VT episodes.

5. Conclusion

This study examines the differences between CAD and non-ischemic DCM patients with ICD. Our results show that patients with DCM exhibit a significantly higher prevalence of VT episodes ($p<0.02$) and a significantly greater variability in the VT initiation pattern ($p<0.01$). The circadian distribution (in a 3 -hour period analysis) of the VT-onset is also different in the two groups: CAD patients exhibit a morning peak: between 9 and 12 a.m. and an afternoon peak (around 6 p.m.), whereas DCM patients show a more uniform distribution during waking hours and very few episodes during the night.
Eventually, no significant differences between CAD and DCM are observed from the analysis of VT-rate, coupling interval, prematurity index. Likewise, the analysis of the EGM signal during the 20 seconds immediately preceding VT onset show no significant differences in the heart-cycle, prevalence of PVC, nor prevalence of paced beats.
This study (based on characterization of EGM, VT-onset and VT circadian distribution) does not define a relationship between observed CAD-DCM differences and underlying CAD-DCM electrogenetic-mechanisms. Nevertheless, our findings suggest different foundations of VT initiation in patients with ischemic versus idiopathic dilated cardiomyopathy.

6. References

Anand K, Aryana A, Cloutier D. (2007) Circadian, daily, and seasonal distributions of ventricular tachyarrhythmias in patients with implantable cardioverter-defibrillators. Am J Cardiol; 100:1134-1138.

Carson PA, O'Connor CM, Miller AB, Anderson S, Belkin R, Neuberg GW et al. (2000) Circadian Rhythm and Sudden Death in Heart Failure. Results from Prospective Randomized Amlodipine Survival Trial. J Am Coll Cardiol; 36:541-546.

Casaleggio A, Rossi P, V Malavasi V, Musso G, Oltrona L. (2008) "Differences between Ventricular Tachyarrhythmias for Patients with Coronary Artery Disease and Dilated Cardiomyopathy." Computers in Cardiology 2008, 35:913-916.

Casaleggio A, Rossi P, Faini A, Guidotto T, Malavasi V, Musso G et al. (2006) Analysis of Implantable Cardioverter Defibrillator Signals for Non Conventional Cardiac Electrical Activity Characterization. Med Biol Eng Comput; 44:45-53.

Chung MK, Pogwizd SM, Miller DP, Cain ME. (1997) Three-Dimensional Mapping of Initiation of Nonsustained Ventricular tachycardia in the Human Heart. Circulation; 95: 2517-2527.

Dorian P. Antiarrhythmic Action of β-Blockers: Potential Mechanisms. (2005) J Cardiovasc Pharmacol Therapeut 10(Supplement I):S15–S22.

Eksik A, Akyol A, Norgaz T, Aksu H, Erdinler I, Cakmak N et al. (2007) Circadian pattern of spontaneous ventricular tachyarrhythmias in patients with implantable cardioverter defibrillators. Med Sci Monit 13:CR412-416.

El-Sherif N, Caref EB, Chinushi M, Restivo M. (1999) Mechanism of Arrhythmogenicity of the Short–Long Cardiac Sequence That Precedes Ventricular Tachyarrhythmias in the Long QT Syndrome. J Am Coll Cardiol 33:1415–1423

Englund A, Behrens S, Wegscheider K, Rowland E, for the European 7219 Jewel Investigators. (1999) Circadian Variation of Malignant Ventricular Arrhythmias in Patients With Ischemic and Nonischemic Heart Disease After Cardioverter Defibrillator Implantation. J Am Coll Cardiol; 34:1560-1568.

Gorenek B, Kudaiberdieva G, Birdane A, Cavusoglu Y, Goktekin O, Unalir A et al. (2006) Importance of initiation pattern of polymorphic ventricular tachycardia in patients with implantable cardioverter defibrillators. Pacing Clin Electrophysiol; 29:48-52.

Henkel DM, Witt BJ. (2006) Ventricular arrhythmias after acute myocardial infarction: A 20-year community study. Am Heart J; 151:806-812.

Himmrich E, Przibille O, Zellerhoff C, Liebrich A, Rosocha S, Andreas K et al. (2003) Proarrhythmic Effect of Pacemaker stimulation in Patients With Implanted Cardioverter-Defibrillators Circulation 108:192-197.

Jayaraj P, Monahan KM. (2005) Sudden cardiac death and the role of device therapy in dilated cardiomyopathy. Curr Heart Fail Rep 2:124-127.

Pogwizd SM, Schlotthaurer K, Li L, et al. (2001). Arrhythmogenesis and contractile dysfunction in heart failure. Circ Res 88: 1159- 1167.

Pogwizd SM and Bers DM. (2004) Cellular Basis of Triggered Arrhythmias in Heart Failure. Trends Cardiovasc Med 14:61–66.

Pogwizd SM, McKenzie JP, Cain ME. (1998) Mechanisms underlying spontaneous and induced ventricular arrhythmias in patients with idiopathic dilated cardiomyopathy. Circulation 98:2404-2414.

Saeed M, Link MS, Mahapatra S, Mouded M, Tzeng D, Jung V et al. (2000) Analysis of intracardiac electrograms showing monomorphic ventricular tachycardia in patients with implantable cardioverter-defibrillators. Am J Cardiol 85:580-587.

Sarter BH, Callans DJ, Gottlieb CD, Schwartzman DS, Marchlinski FE. (1998) Implantable Defibrillator Diagnostic Storage Capabilities: Evolution, Current Status and Future Utilization. Pacing Clin Electrophysiol 21:1287-1298.

Sweeney MO, Ruetz LL, Belk P, Mullen TJ, Johnson JW, Sheldon T. (2007) Bradycardia pacing-induced short-long-short sequences at the onset of ventricular tachyarrhythmias: a possible mechanism of proarrhythmia? J Am Coll Cardiol 50:614-622.

Taneda K, Aizawa Y on behalf of the Japanese ICD study group. (2001) Absence of a Morning Peak in Ventricular Tachycardia and Fibrillation Events in Nonischemic Heart Disease: Analysis of Therapies by Implantable Cardioverter Defibrillators. Pacing Clin Electrophysiol 24:1602-1606.

Taylor E, Berger R, Hummel JD, Dinerman JL, Kenknight B, Arria AM et al. (2000) Analysis of the pattern of initiation of sustained ventricular arrhythmias in patients with implantable defibrillators. J Cardiovasc. Electrophysiol 11:719-726.

Vlay LC, Vlay SC. (1997) Pacing induced ventricular fibrillation in internal cardioverter defibrillator patients: a new form of proarrhythmia. Pacing Clin Electrophysiol 20:132-133

Part 2

Prediction, Prevention, and Management of Cardiovascular Events

5

Prediction of Ventricular Arrhythmias in Patients at Risk of Sudden Cardiac Death

K.H. Haugaa, J.P. Amlie and T. Edvardsen
Oslo University Hospital, Rikshospitalet, Oslo and University of Oslo, Norway

1. Introduction

Sudden cardiac deaths remain the major cause of mortality in the western world. Ventricular arrhythmia due to ischemic heart disease is the most frequent cause of sudden cardiac death. In patients >35 years of age, ischemic heart disease is the most frequent cause of ventricular arrhythmias. In patients <35 years of age, inherited cardiac diseases play a significant role in sudden cardiac death. Prediction of who will experience a life-threatening ventricular arrhythmia is a major challenge in current cardiology.
An implantable cardioverter defibrillator (ICD) provides efficient preventive treatment for ventricular arrhythmias and sudden death and is implanted in patients at risk. However, risk stratification of ventricular arrhythmias is insufficient and the majority of patients dying suddenly have not been evaluated for ICD therapy.
Patients after myocardial infarction are at high risk for cardiac arrhythmic events and sudden cardiac death (Zipes, 2006). Currently, LV ejection fraction (EF) is the primary parameter used to select patients for ICD therapy after a myocardial infarction. Impaired EF is shown to be a marker of increased cardiovascular mortality and sudden cardiac death. However, EF has relatively low sensitivity to detect arrhythmic risk (Buxton, 2007). A number of other diagnostic tests have been proposed to improve the accuracy for selection of patients for ICD therapy. Currently available data, however, are not adequate to routinely recommend additional risk-stratification methods for selection of patients for ICD therapy (Passman, 2007).
The presence of myocardial scar forms the substrate for malignant arrhythmias (Zipes, 1998). Heterogeneity in scar tissue may create areas of slow conduction that generate the substrate for ventricular arrhythmia post-myocardial infarction (Verma, 2005). Electrical dispersion, including both activation time and refractoriness, in infarcted tissue is a known arrhythmogenic factor, (Endresen, 1987; Han, 1964; Janse, 1989; Vassallo, 1988). Electrical abnormalities may lead to distorted myocardial function (Nagueh, 2008). Therefore, regional differences in electrical properties may cause heterogeneity of myocardial contraction which can be recognized as myocardial dyssynchrony (Yu, 2003).
In this report, a novel echocardiographic method will be presented in order to evaluate the cardiac contractility pattern in patients at increased risk of life-threatening arrhythmias.

2. Modern echocardiographic modalities

Better echocardiographic tools for more accurate assessment of ventricular function have been developed during the last 2 decades. Minor degrees of myocardial contraction heterogeneity and contraction dyssynchrony can be demonstrated by these modern echocardiographic techniques (Reisner, 2004; Yu, 2007). One way to discover subtle wall motion abnormalities caused by electrical heterogeneity would be to use strain echocardiography (Edvardsen, 2002b). The introduction of strain echocardiography has made it possible to accurately perform quantitative and objective measures of regional ventricular function by measuring regional contraction by strain. Strain can accurately quantify timing and deformation of regional myocardial function (Edvardsen, 2002a; Reisner, 2004; Voigt, 2003).

Currently, visual assessment of regional myocardial function from 2-D image is the standard echocardiographic method to assess ventricular function in daily clinical practice. Visual assessment has had that position since the introduction of 2-D echocardiography. This method has also been established as a clinically important tool in detecting regional ventricular function, but has limited ability to detect more subtle changes in function and changes in timing of myocardial motion throughout systole and diastole. Strain echocardiographic technique may be used to accurately assess timing and function of myocardial contraction in patients with increased risk of ventricular arrhythmias. The hypotheses that echocardiography can contribute to arrhythmic risk assessment is based on the assumption that arrhythmogenic electrical abnormalities will lead to mechanical alterations which can be assessed by strain echocardiography.

2.1 Use of strain echocardiography for prediction of ventricular arrhythmias

We have recently reported that strain echocardiography can be used as a novel risk predictor of ventricular arrhythmias in patients with the long QT syndrome (Haugaa, 2009; Haugaa, 2010a). The long QT syndrome has traditionally been regarded as a purely electrical disease. Sporadic reports have indicated, however, that the electrical alterations may lead to mechanical consequences (De Ferrari, 2009; Nador, 1991). In our publications, we could show by modern echocardiographic techniques that subtle contraction heterogeneity was present in patients with the long QT syndrome, possibly due to electrical abnormalities. Therefore, these echocardiographic techniques were able to detect subtle changes in myocardial function. Furthermore, we could associate mechanical dispersion to ventricular arrhythmias in patients with arrhythmogenic right ventricular cardiomyopathy (Sarvari, 2011). Contraction heterogeneity defined as mechanical dispersion was a marker of arrhythmias in these patients and could help risk stratification of arrhythmias in so far asymptomatic mutation carriers. In a recent paper, we investigated if contraction heterogeneity due to fibrosis in infarcted myocardial tissue leads to mechanical dispersion in patients after myocardial infarction (Haugaa, 2010b). These results are briefly presented below. We presumed that the mechanical dispersion reflected electrical heterogeneity. We investigated if mechanical dispersion can predict ventricular arrhythmias in patients with risk of ventricular arrhythmias. Furthermore, we investigated if global strain by echocardiography is a better marker of arrhythmias than EF in patients after myocardial infarction.

3. Study of 85 post MI patients with an ICD

We prospectively investigated 85 post-MI patients fulfilling indications for ICD therapy. All patients had prior myocardial infarction and indication for ICD therapy according to primary or secondary prevention criteria. Arrhythmic events, defined as ventricular arrhythmias that required appropriate anti tachycardia pacing or shock from the ICD, were recorded. During 2.3 years of follow up, 45% of the ICD patients experienced one or more episodes with sustained ventricular tachycardia or ventricular fibrillation requiring appropriate ICD therapy (anti tachycardia pacing or shock) while 55% had no sustained arrhythmia during follow up.

Speckle tracking technique by strain echocardiography was used to assess the contraction duration in each of the 16 left ventricular segments (Figure 1). Mechanical dispersion was calculated as the standard deviation from contraction durations the 16 left ventricular segments. Global left ventricular strain was obtained by averaging all segmental values for maximum shortening in a 16 segment model.

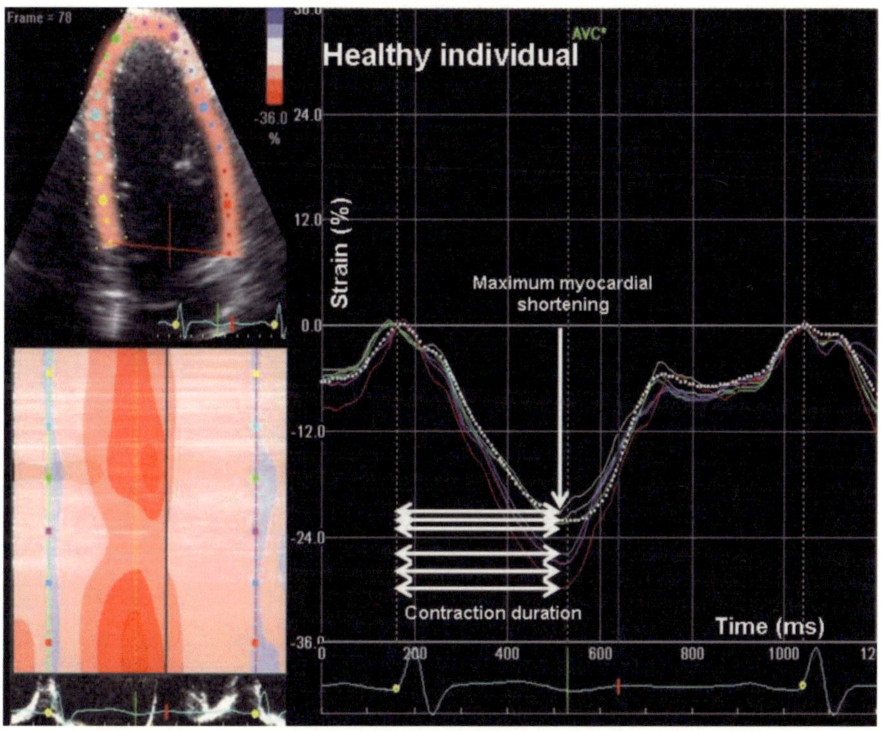

Fig. 1. Speckle tracking longitudinal strain curves from 6 segments in apical 4 chamber view from a healthy individual with synchronous ECG recording below. Segment contraction (shortening) starts during QRS and reaches a maximum myocardial shortening (white vertical arrow) at the end of the ECG T-wave. (Modified from *JACC Cardiovasc Imaging* 2010 March;**3**(3):247-56).

The study showed that mechanical dispersion was significantly more pronounced in those with arrhythmias compared to those without (Fig 2). Furthermore, mechanical dispersion was a strong and independent predictor of arrhythmias requiring ICD therapy.

Survival analyses showed that ICD patients with mechanical dispersion > 70ms showed more frequent arrhythmic events than ICD patients with dispersion < 70ms (Fig 3).

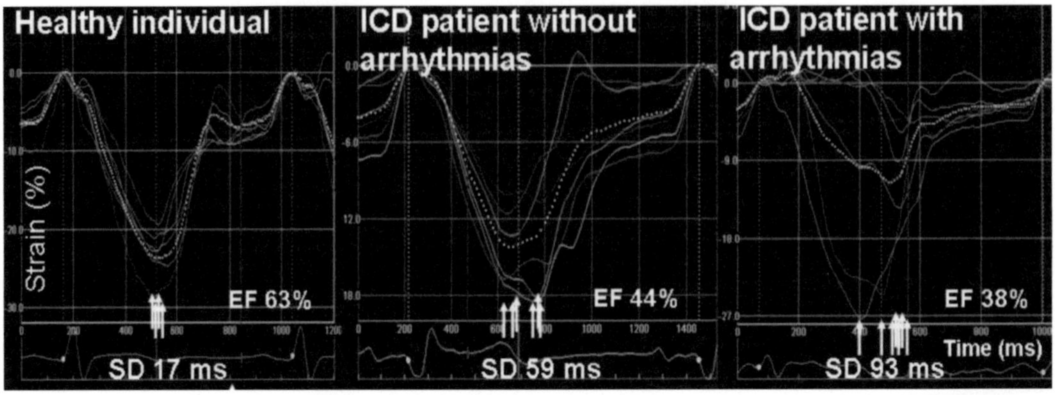

Fig. 2. Strain curves from a healthy individual (left panel), a post MI patient with arrhythmias (mid panel) and a post MI patient with recurrent arrhythmias (right panel). White arrows indicate timing of maximum myocardial shortening. The post MI patient with recurrent arrhythmias (right panel) has the most dispersed timing in myocardial contraction and thereby most pronounced mechanical dispersion. (Modified from *JACC Cardiovasc Imaging* 2010 March;**3**(3):247-56).

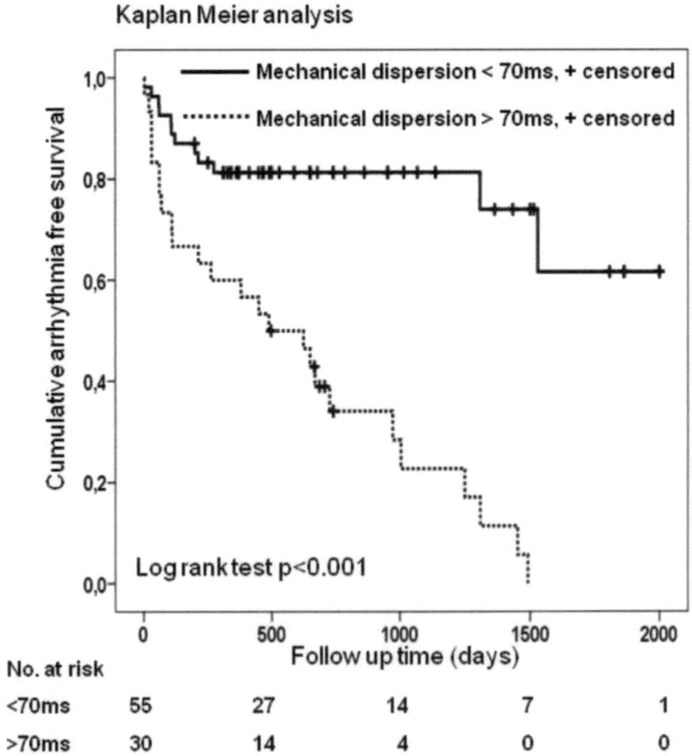

Fig. 3. Kaplan Meier analyses of 85 patients after myocardial infarction with ICD. Patients with mechanical dispersion > 70 ms have higher rate of arrhythmic events during follow up compared to patients with mechanical dispersion < 70 ms. (Modified from *JACC Cardiovasc Imaging* 2010 March;**3**(3):247-56).

In ICD patients with EF > 35%, mechanical dispersion was more pronounced in those who experienced arrhythmia compared to those without. Global strain showed better left ventricular function in those without recorded arrhythmias, while EF did not differ.
The results of the study showed that increased heterogeneity of myocardial contraction measured by strain echocardiography predicted cardiac arrhythmias better than current risk stratification tools. This novel method may improve risk stratification of cardiac arrhythmias and help the clinician to select patients for ICD therapy.

4. Electromechanical interactions

There is ample evidence from different cardiac disease models, including heart failure (Tomaselli, 2004), ischemia (Han, 1964) and infarction (Spragg, 2005; Vassallo, 1988) that increases in dispersion of conduction velocity result in susceptibility to arrhythmias (Spragg, 2005; Tomaselli, 2004). These electrical abnormalities will presumptively lead to changes in myocardial function. Assessing the extent of electrical dispersion in the individual patient has so far been difficult (Tomaselli, 2004). These findings support the idea that tissue heterogeneity in and around scarred myocardium lead to a dispersed myocardial contraction and is associated with risk of arrhythmic events.
Earlier echocardiographic studies have observed that an EF of ≤40% serves as the threshold for identifying high-risk individuals (Bigger, Jr., 1984; Greenberg, 1984). However, EF has reduced sensitivity in predicting sudden death (Buxton, 2007; Stecker, 2006). Speckle based strain has shown to be a robust technique for assessment of LV function and a recent study has demonstrated that speckle tracking strain is superior to EF for assessment of myocardial function post-myocardial infarction (Gjesdal, 2008). Global strain discriminated between those with and without arrhythmic events in post-MI patients with EF > 35%. This finding suggests that global strain might become a useful tool for risk stratification in post-myocardial infarction patients with relatively preserved LV function. Future trials should investigate if mechanical dispersion and global strain can be used to select additional patients for ICD therapy among the majority of patients after myocardial infarction with relatively preserved EF in whom current ICD indications fail.

5. Risk assessment of ventricular arrhythmias in patients with arrhythmogenic right ventricular cardiomyopathy

Arrhythmogenic right ventricular cardiomyopathy is an inheritable, chronic and progressive cardiomyopathy and is one of the leading causes of sudden unexpected cardiac death in previously healthy young individuals (Sen-Chowdhry, 2010a; Thiene, 1988). Prevalence has been estimated to be at least 1 in 1000 (Sen-Chowdhry, 2010a).
Recent molecular genetic reports have revealed arrhythmogenic right ventricular cardiomyopathy as mainly a desmosomal disease (Xu, 2010). Mutations in one of the 5 desmosomal or 3 extra desmosomal genes so far identified, lead to progressive loss of myocytes, followed by fibro-fatty replacement. Penetrance is age and gender dependent and the progressive clinical picture is highly variable (Dalal, 2006).
Four clinical stages have been documented: An early concealed phase, overt electrical disorder, isolated right heart failure (Fig 4a), and biventricular pump failure (Fig 4b) (Basso, 1996; Sen-Chowdhry, 2007; Sen-Chowdhry, 2010a). Importantly, life-threatening arrhythmias can occur with only discrete or even absent myocardial structural changes (Sen-

Chowdhry, 2010b). Risk stratification of ventricular arrhythmias and sudden cardiac death is therefore challenging.

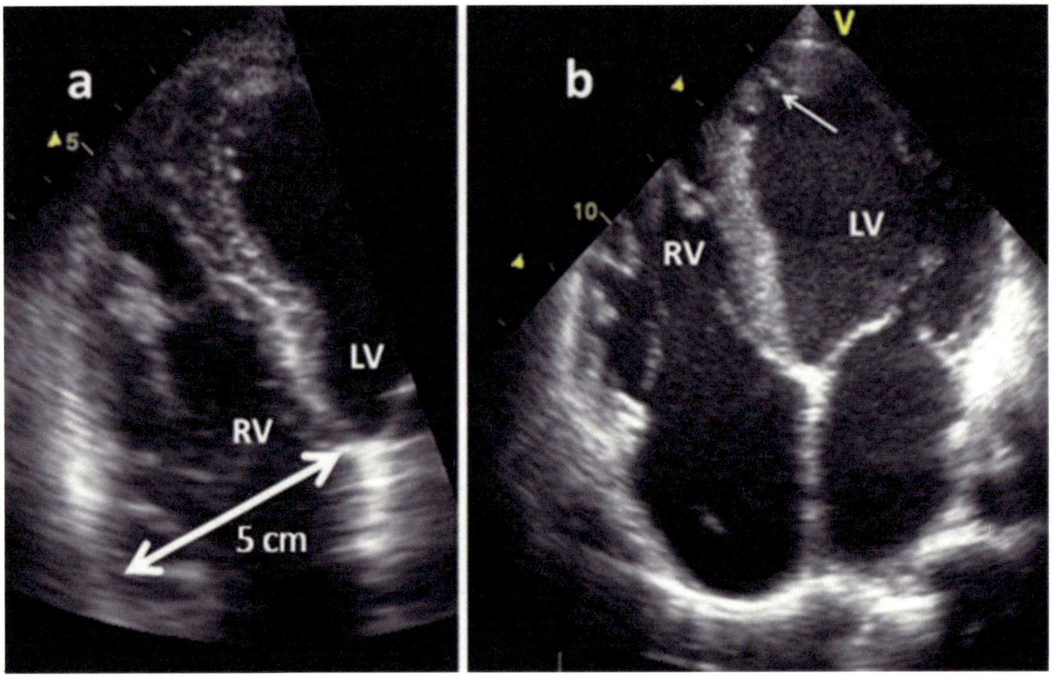

Fig. 4. Echocardiographic pictures of 2 patients with arrhythmogenic right ventricular cardiomyopathy.
A) left panel: classical right sided affection with dilatation (5 cm diameter, white arrow) and wall thinning of the right ventricle. The ICD lead is visible in the right ventricle.
B) right panel: Affection of both right and left ventricle in a patient with arrhythmogenic right ventricular cardiomyopathy. The right ventricle is dilated and with visible ICD lead. Furthermore, the left ventricle is dilated and shows apical affection of the myocardial wall (arrow).

Mechanisms of arrhythmias in early stages of arrhythmogenic right ventricular cardiomyopathy are probably due to dysfunction of desmosomal proteins and disturbed cell to cell coupling (Saffitz, 2009). In later stages of arrhythmogenic right ventricular cardiomyopathy when structural abnormalities in the myocardium have developed, reentrant ventricular arrhythmias can occur in tissue with fibro fatty replacement. Therefore, electrical conduction delay with consequent electrical dispersion has been suggested as an important mechanism of ventricular arrhythmias (Amlie, 1997; Turrini, 2001).
In a recent study we investigated if arrhythmogenic right ventricular cardiomyopathy patients had cardiac contraction heterogeneity assessed as mechanical dispersion and if contraction heterogeneity was associated with susceptibility to ventricular arrhythmias

(Sarvari, 2011). Furthermore, we investigated if mechanical dispersion was present in arrhythmogenic right ventricular cardiomyopathy mutation carriers in early stages of the disease where no structural alterations were visible.

Mechanical dispersion and strain in right and left ventricle were assessed in 36 arrhythmogenic right ventricular cardiomyopathy patients, in 23 asymptomatic arrhythmogenic right ventricular cardiomyopathy mutation carriers and in 30 healthy individuals. All 36 arrhythmogenic right ventricular cardiomyopathy patients had experienced ventricular arrhythmias either as aborted cardiac arrest or as documented sustained ventricular tachycardia and fulfilled 2010 International Task Force criteria (Marcus, 2010). They were treated with ICD in addition to medical anti arrhythmic therapy. The 23 asymptomatic mutation carriers were family members of the arrhythmogenic right ventricular cardiomyopathy patients and were diagnosed by cascade genetic screening.

Peak systolic myocardial strain by 2D speckle tracking echocardiography was assessed in 16 left ventricular segments and averaged to left ventricular global longitudinal strain in arrhythmogenic right ventricular cardiomyopathy patients. Additionally, peak systolic strain from 3 right ventricular free wall segments was averaged as a measure of right ventricular function (RV strain) (Fig 5). Contraction duration was measured as time from onset R on ECG to maximum LV and right ventricular shortening by strain. Standard deviation of contraction duration was calculated as mechanical dispersion, in a 16 left ventricular segments and a 6 right ventricular segments model.

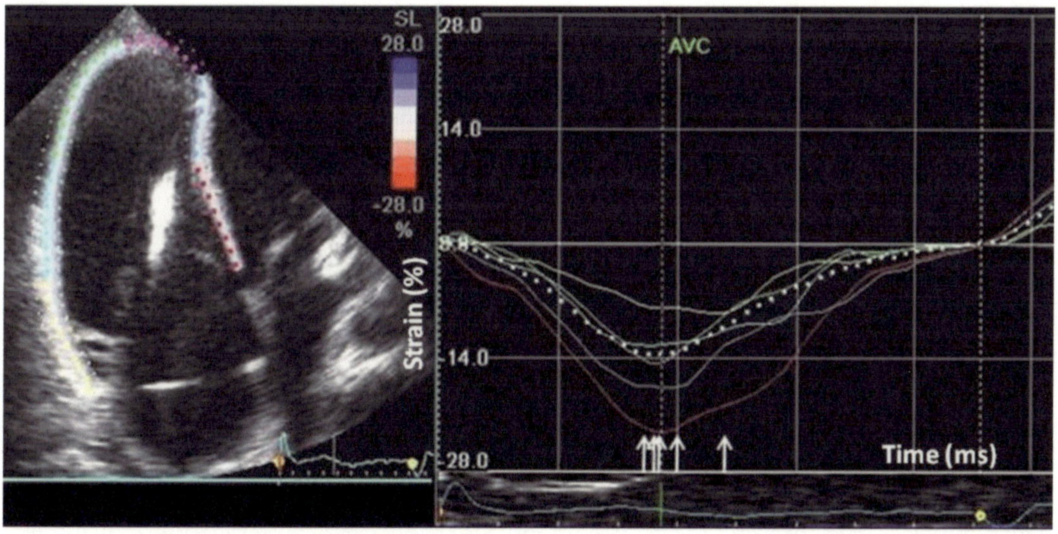

Fig. 5. Strain curves in an patient with arrhythmogenic right ventricular cardiomyopathy. Strain curves from a dilated right ventricle from apical 4 chamber view. Vertical arrows indicate the timing of maximum myocardial shortening in each right ventricular segment and are consistent with pronounced right ventricular mechanical dispersion.

Mechanical dispersion was more pronounced in arrhythmogenic right ventricular cardiomyopathy patients with arrhythmias in right and left ventricle compared to asymptomatic mutation carriers and healthy individuals (Table 1). Importantly, mechanical dispersion was more pronounced in asymptomatic mutation carriers compared to healthy individuals in both right and left ventricle, indicating sub clinical ventricular involvement. Right and left ventricular strains were reduced in arrhythmogenic right ventricular cardiomyopathy patients compared to asymptomatic mutation carriers and healthy individuals (Table 1). Reduced right and left ventricular strains were significantly correlated in arrhythmogenic right ventricular cardiomyopathy patients, indicating biventricular disease. Right and left ventricular function in asymptomatic mutation carriers were within normal range, but significantly reduced compared to healthy individuals.

	Healthy individuals (n=30)	Asymptomatic mutation carriers (n=23)	ARVC patients with arrhythmias (n=36)	P
EF (%)	64±5	63±4	57±14*	<0.01
LV strain (%)	-23±2	-20±2*	-16±5*,**	<0.001
RV strain (%)	-28±5	-24±5*	-19±7*,**	<0.001
LV Dispersion (ms)	22±8	42±13*	64±25*,**	<0.001
RV Dispersion (ms)	15±8	33±20*	53±25*,**	<0.001

Table 1. Echocardiographic results in 36 ARVC patients, 23 asymptomatic ARVC mutation carriers and 30 healthy individuals.
Mean±SD. Right column shows P-values for ANOVA test. Flags for significance are obtained from the post hoc pair-wise comparison using the Bonferroni correction. *$p<0.05$ compared with healthy individuals. **$p<0.01$ compared with asymptomatic mutation carriers. ANOVA, analysis of variance; EF, ejection fraction; RV, right ventricular; LV, left ventricular.

Risk stratification of ventricular arrhythmias in so far asymptomatic arrhythmogenic right ventricular cardiomyopathy mutation carriers is difficult. This report demonstrated that mechanical dispersion was closely related to ventricular arrhythmias in patients with arrhythmogenic right ventricular cardiomyopathy. Increased mechanical dispersion in both ventricles was present in asymptomatic mutation carriers, indicating sub clinical myocardial alterations. Importantly, pronounced mechanical dispersion was also present in individuals who had experienced arrhythmias in the early stages of arrhythmogenic right ventricular cardiomyopathy and in whom no structural alterations assessed by conventional echocardiography and magnetic resonance imaging could be assessed. These findings suggest that mechanical dispersion may be a marker of arrhythmic events and help risk stratification in so far asymptomatic arrhythmogenic right ventricular cardiomyopathy mutation carriers. Mechanical dispersion and myocardial strains demonstrated subclinical myocardial involvement in these individuals. Longitudinal follow up studies are required to assess if these methods can provide added value in arrhythmia risk stratification in asymptomatic arrhythmogenic right ventricular cardiomyopathy mutation carriers.

Furthermore, this paper demonstrated frequent and early left ventricular involvement in arrhythmogenic right ventricular cardiomyopathy which supported recent reports of arrhythmogenic right ventricular cardiomyopathy as a biventricular disease (Kjaergaard, 2007). Biventricular impairment is probably a result of biventricular arrhythmogenic right ventricular cardiomyopathy affection, but mutual dependency of right and left ventricular hemodynamics may be considered. In patients with overt arrhythmogenic right ventricular cardiomyopathy, strain echocardiography may be a useful tool for quantification of right and left sided myocardial dysfunction.

6. Comparisons of mechanical dispersion in patients after myocardial infarction and in patients with arrhythmogenic right ventricular cardiomyopathy

Mechanical dispersion has been demonstrated in arrhythmogenic right ventricular cardiomyopathy patients and in post-myocardial infarction patients and has been shown to be a marker of recurrent ventricular arrhythmias in both conditions. The mechanisms for arrhythmias in arrhythmogenic right ventricular cardiomyopathy and in infarcted myocardial tissue are different, but have similarities regarding electrical dispersion. In arrhythmogenic right ventricular cardiomyopathy patients, mechanisms of arrhythmias are probably stage dependent, but electrical dispersion has been considered to be of importance in early and later stages of the disease (Amlie, 1997; Turrini, 2001). In post-MI patients delayed start of ventricular activation in scarred myocardium leads to a dispersed recovery of excitability (Vassallo, 1988), finally resulting in dispersed electrical repolarization. One might therefore speculate that electrical dispersion may be regarded as the final common pathway of arrhythmia mechanism in both conditions.

The extent of mechanical dispersion appeared most pronounced in post-myocardial infarction patients. This difference was probably a result of the concomitant contractile impairment in infarcted tissue which was more pronounced compared to presence of fibrosis in arrhythmogenic right ventricular cardiomyopathy. Myocardial function was significantly impaired in post-myocardial infarction patients compared to arrhythmogenic right ventricular cardiomyopathy patients. Contractile impairment will pronounce mechanical dispersion. The ranges and values of mechanical dispersion which are related to increased arrhythmic risk will therefore not necessarily be interchangeable between different myocardial diseases.

7. Future risk assessment of ventricular arrhythmias and additional patient entities

The most important patient group for further risk assessment of ventricular arrhythmias are patients after myocardial infarction representing the largest cohort of individuals at risk. Future trials should investigate if mechanical dispersion and global strain can be used to select additional patients for ICD therapy among the majority of post-myocardial infarction patients with relatively preserved EF in whom current ICD indications fail. Furthermore, there are several large groups of patients who are at risk of ventricular arrhythmias on a non-ischemic basis, i.e. patients with idiopathic dilated cardiomyopathies, other cardiomyopathies and patients with congenital heart disease. It is of great concern that EF is currently the only parameter to select patients with idiopathic dilated cardiomyopathy for ICD therapy. There is emerging awareness of the insufficiency of EF to predict ventricular arrhythmias in these patients and further risk stratification tools are urgently needed. Mechanical dispersion may reflect the electrical dispersion and represent a fundamental arrhythmogenic factor. Furthermore, mechanical dispersion has been shown to predict arrhythmias independently of EF. Mechanical dispersion may therefore have the potential to be introduced as an additional tool in arrhythmic risk stratification in other groups of patients.

8. Conclusion

In summary, mechanical dispersion has been shown to predict ventricular arrhythmias in post-myocardial infarction patients and in patients with arrhythmogenic right ventricular cardiomyopathy and the long QT syndrome. This principle may therefore be a valuable supplement in evaluating patients at risk independently of EF. Mechanical dispersion and global strain may be useful for including more patients for ICD therapy after myocardial infarction.

9. References

Amlie, JP. (1997). Dispersion of repolarization. A basic electrophysiological mechanism behind malignant arrhythmias. *Eur Heart J,* Vol. 18, No. 8, pp. 1200-1202.

Basso, C, Thiene, G, Corrado, D, Angelini, A, Nava, A, & Valente, M. (1996). Arrhythmogenic right ventricular cardiomyopathy. Dysplasia, dystrophy, or myocarditis? *Circulation,* Vol. 94, No. 5, pp. 983-991.

Bigger, JT, Jr., Fleiss, JL, Kleiger, R, Miller, JP, & Rolnitzky, LM. (1984). The relationships among ventricular arrhythmias, left ventricular dysfunction, and mortality in the 2 years after myocardial infarction. *Circulation,* Vol. 69, No. 2, pp. 250-258.

Buxton, AE, Lee, KL, Hafley, GE, Pires, LA, Fisher, JD, Gold, MR, Josephson, ME, Lehmann, MH, & Prystowsky, EN. (2007). Limitations of ejection fraction for prediction of sudden death risk in patients with coronary artery disease: lessons from the MUSTT study. *Journal of the American College of Cardiology,* Vol. 50, No. 12, pp. 1150-1157.

Dalal, D, James, C, Devanagondi, R, Tichnell, C, Tucker, A, Prakasa, K, Spevak, PJ, Bluemke, DA, Abraham, T, Russell, SD, Calkins, H, & Judge, DP. (2006). Penetrance of mutations in plakophilin-2 among families with arrhythmogenic right ventricular dysplasia/cardiomyopathy. *J.Am.Coll.Cardiol.,* Vol. 48, No. 7, pp. 1416-1424.

De Ferrari, GM,Schwartz, PJ. (2009). Long QT syndrome, a purely electrical disease? Not anymore. *Eur Heart J,* Vol. 30, No. 3, pp. 253-255.

Edvardsen, T, Gerber, BL, Garot, J, Bluemke, DA, Lima, JA, & Smiseth, OA. (2002a). Quantitative assessment of intrinsic regional myocardial deformation by Doppler strain rate echocardiography in humans: validation against three-dimensional tagged magnetic resonance imaging. *Circulation*, Vol. 106, No. 1, pp. 50-56.

Edvardsen, T, Urheim, S, Skulstad, H, Steine, K, Ihlen, H, & Smiseth, OA. (2002b). Quantification of left ventricular systolic function by tissue Doppler echocardiography: added value of measuring pre- and postejection velocities in ischemic myocardium. *Circulation*, Vol. 105, No. 17, pp. 2071-2077.

Endresen, K, Amlie, JP, Forfang, K, Simonsen, S, & Jensen, O. (1987). Monophasic action potentials in patients with coronary artery disease: reproducibility and electrical restitution and conduction at different stimulation rates. *Cardiovasc Res.*, Vol. 21, No. 9, pp. 696-702.

Gjesdal, O, Helle-Valle, T, Hopp, E, Lunde, K, Vartdal, T, Aakhus, S, Smith, HJ, Ihlen, H, & Edvardsen, T. (2008). Noninvasive Separation of Large, Medium, and Small Myocardial Infarcts in Survivors of Reperfused ST-Elevation Myocardial Infarction: A Comprehensive Tissue Doppler and Speckle-Tracking Echocardiography Study. *Circ Cardiovasc Imaging*, Vol. 1, pp. 189-196.

Greenberg, H, McMaster, P, & Dwyer, EM, Jr. (1984). Left ventricular dysfunction after acute myocardial infarction: results of a prospective multicenter study. *Journal of the American College of Cardiology*, Vol. 4, No. 5, pp. 867-874.

Han, J,Moe, GK. (1964). Nonuniform recovery of excitability in ventricular muscle. *Circulation Research*, Vol. 12, pp. 44-60.

Haugaa, KH, Amlie, JP, Berge, KE, Leren, TP, Smiseth, OA, & Edvardsen, T. (2010a). Transmural differences in myocardial contraction in long-QT syndrome: mechanical consequences of ion channel dysfunction. *Circulation*, Vol. 122, No. 14, pp. 1355-1363.

Haugaa, KH, Edvardsen, T, Leren, TP, Gran, JM, Smiseth, OA, & Amlie, JP. (2009). Left ventricular mechanical dispersion by tissue Doppler imaging: a novel approach for identifying high-risk individuals with long QT syndrome. *Eur Heart J*, Vol. 30, No. 3, pp. 330-337.

Haugaa, KH, Smedsrud, MK, Steen, T, Kongsgaard, E, Loennechen, JP, Skjaerpe, T, Voigt, JU, Willems, R, Smith, G, Smiseth, OA, Amlie, JP, & Edvardsen, T. (2010b). Mechanical dispersion assessed by myocardial strain in patients after myocardial infarction for risk prediction of ventricular arrhythmia. *JACC.Cardiovasc Imaging*, Vol. 3, No. 3, pp. 247-256.

Janse, MJ,Wit, AL. (1989). Electrophysiological mechanisms of ventricular arrhythmias resulting from myocardial ischemia and infarction. *Physiol Rev.*, Vol. 69, No. 4, pp. 1049-1169.

Kjaergaard, J, Hastrup, SJ, Sogaard, P, Chen, X, Bay, NH, Kober, L, Kjaer, A, & Hassager, C. (2007). Advanced quantitative echocardiography in arrhythmogenic right ventricular cardiomyopathy. *J Am Soc.Echocardiogr.*, Vol. 20, No. 1, pp. 27-35.

Marcus, FI, McKenna, WJ, Sherrill, D, Basso, C, Bauce, B, Bluemke, DA, Calkins, H, Corrado, D, Cox, MG, Daubert, JP, Fontaine, G, Gear, K, Hauer, R, Nava, A, Picard, MH, Protonotarios, N, Saffitz, JE, Sanborn, DM, Steinberg, JS, Tandri, H, Thiene, G, Towbin, JA, Tsatsopoulou, A, Wichter, T, & Zareba, W. (2010). Diagnosis of arrhythmogenic right ventricular cardiomyopathy/dysplasia:

proposed modification of the task force criteria. *Circulation,* Vol. 121, No. 13, pp. 1533-1541.

Nador, F, Beria, G, De Ferrari, GM, Stramba-Badiale, M, Locati, EH, Lotto, A, & Schwartz, PJ. (1991). Unsuspected echocardiographic abnormality in the long QT syndrome. Diagnostic, prognostic, and pathogenetic implications. *Circulation,* Vol. 84, No. 4, pp. 1530-1542.

Nagueh, SF. (2008). Mechanical dyssynchrony in congestive heart failure: diagnostic and therapeutic implications. *J Am Coll Cardiol,* Vol. 51, No. 1, pp. 18-22.

Olsson, S. B., Shiwen, Y., and Amlie, J. P. Dispersion of repolarisation. State of the Art. Olsson, S. B., Shiwen, Y., and Amlie, J. P. 2000. New York 10504, USA, Futura Publishing Company.

Ref Type: Book, Whole

Passman, R,Kadish, A. (2007). Sudden death prevention with implantable devices. *Circulation,* Vol. 116, No. 5, pp. 561-571.

Reisner, SA, Lysyansky, P, Agmon, Y, Mutlak, D, Lessick, J, & Friedman, Z. (2004). Global longitudinal strain: a novel index of left ventricular systolic function. *Journal of the American Society of Echocardiography,* Vol. 17, No. 6, pp. 630-633.

Saffitz, JE. (2009). Arrhythmogenic cardiomyopathy and abnormalities of cell-to-cell coupling. *Heart Rhythm,* Vol. 6, No. 8 Suppl, pp. S62-S65.

Sarvari, SI, Haugaa, KH, Anfinsen, OG, Leren, TP, Smiseth, OA, Kongsgaard, E, Amlie, JP, & Edvardsen, T. (2011). Right ventricular mechanical dispersion is related to malignant arrhythmias: a study of patients with arrhythmogenic right ventricular cardiomyopathy and subclinical right ventricular dysfunction. *Eur.Heart J.*

Sen-Chowdhry, S, Morgan, RD, Chambers, JC, & McKenna, WJ. (2010a). Arrhythmogenic cardiomyopathy: etiology, diagnosis, and treatment. *Annu.Rev.Med.,* Vol. 61, pp. 233-253.

Sen-Chowdhry, S, Morgan, RD, Chambers, JC, & McKenna, WJ. (2010b). Arrhythmogenic cardiomyopathy: etiology, diagnosis, and treatment. *Annu.Rev.Med,* Vol. 61, pp. 233-253.

Sen-Chowdhry, S, Syrris, P, Ward, D, Asimaki, A, Sevdalis, E, & McKenna, WJ. (2007). Clinical and genetic characterization of families with arrhythmogenic right ventricular dysplasia/cardiomyopathy provides novel insights into patterns of disease expression. *Circulation,* Vol. 115, No. 13, pp. 1710-1720.

Spragg, DD, Akar, FG, Helm, RH, Tunin, RS, Tomaselli, GF, & Kass, DA. (2005). Abnormal conduction and repolarization in late-activated myocardium of dyssynchronously contracting hearts. *Cardiovascular Research,* Vol. 67, No. 1, pp. 77-86.

Stecker, EC, Vickers, C, Waltz, J, Socoteanu, C, John, BT, Mariani, R, McAnulty, JH, Gunson, K, Jui, J, & Chugh, SS. (2006). Population-based analysis of sudden cardiac death with and without left ventricular systolic dysfunction: two-year findings from the Oregon Sudden Unexpected Death Study. *Journal of the American College of Cardiology,* Vol. 47, No. 6, pp. 1161-1166.

Thiene, G, Nava, A, Corrado, D, Rossi, L, & Pennelli, N. (1988). Right ventricular cardiomyopathy and sudden death in young people. *N.Engl.J.Med.*, Vol. 318, No. 3, pp. 129-133.

Tomaselli, GF,Zipes, DP. (2004). What causes sudden death in heart failure? *Circulation Research,* Vol. 95, No. 8, pp. 754-763.

Turrini, P, Corrado, D, Basso, C, Nava, A, Bauce, B, & Thiene, G. (2001). Dispersion of ventricular depolarization-repolarization: a noninvasive marker for risk stratification in arrhythmogenic right ventricular cardiomyopathy. *Circulation,* Vol. 103, No. 25, pp. 3075-3080.

Vassallo, JA, Cassidy, DM, Kindwall, KE, Marchlinski, FE, & Josephson, ME. (1988). Nonuniform recovery of excitability in the left ventricle. *Circulation,* Vol. 78, No. 6, pp. 1365-1372.

Verma, A, Marrouche, NF, Schweikert, RA, Saliba, W, Wazni, O, Cummings, J, bdul-Karim, A, Bhargava, M, Burkhardt, JD, Kilicaslan, F, Martin, DO, & Natale, A. (2005). Relationship between successful ablation sites and the scar border zone defined by substrate mapping for ventricular tachycardia post-myocardial infarction. *Journal of Cardiovascular Electrophysiology,* Vol. 16, No. 5, pp. 465-471.

Voigt, JU, Exner, B, Schmiedehausen, K, Huchzermeyer, C, Reulbach, U, Nixdorff, U, Platsch, G, Kuwert, T, Daniel, WG, & Flachskampf, FA. (2003). Strain-rate imaging during dobutamine stress echocardiography provides objective evidence of inducible ischemia. *Circulation,* Vol. 107, No. 16, pp. 2120-2126.

Xu, T, Yang, Z, Vatta, M, Rampazzo, A, Beffagna, G, Pilichou, K, Scherer, SE, Saffitz, J, Kravitz, J, Zareba, W, Danieli, GA, Lorenzon, A, Nava, A, Bauce, B, Thiene, G, Basso, C, Calkins, H, Gear, K, Marcus, F, & Towbin, JA. (2010). Compound and digenic heterozygosity contributes to arrhythmogenic right ventricular cardiomyopathy. *Journal of the American College of Cardiology,* Vol. 55, No. 6, pp. 587-597.

Yu, CM, Lin, H, Zhang, Q, & Sanderson, JE. (2003). High prevalence of left ventricular systolic and diastolic asynchrony in patients with congestive heart failure and normal QRS duration. *Heart,* Vol. 89, No. 1, pp. 54-60.

Yu, CM, Sanderson, JE, Marwick, TH, & Oh, JK. (2007). Tissue Doppler imaging a new prognosticator for cardiovascular diseases. *J Am.Coll.Cardiol.,* Vol. 49, No. 19, pp. 1903-1914.

Zipes, DP, Camm, AJ, Borggrefe, M, Buxton, AE, Chaitman, B, Fromer, M, Gregoratos, G, Klein, G, Moss, AJ, Myerburg, RJ, Priori, SG, Quinones, MA, Roden, DM, Silka, MJ, Tracy, C, Smith, SC, Jr., Jacobs, AK, Adams, CD, Antman, EM, Anderson, JL, Hunt, SA, Halperin, JL, Nishimura, R, Ornato, JP, Page, RL, Riegel, B, Priori, SG, Blanc, JJ, Budaj, A, Camm, AJ, Dean, V, Deckers, JW, Despres, C, Dickstein, K, Lekakis, J, McGregor, K, Metra, M, Morais, J, Osterspey, A, Tamargo, JL, & Zamorano, JL. (2006). ACC/AHA/ESC 2006 guidelines for management of patients with ventricular arrhythmias and the prevention of sudden cardiac death: a report of the American College of Cardiology/American Heart Association Task Force and the European Society of Cardiology Committee for Practice Guidelines (Writing Committee to Develop Guidelines for Management of Patients With Ventricular Arrhythmias and the Prevention of Sudden Cardiac Death). *Journal of the American College of Cardiology,* Vol. 48, No. 5, pp. e247-e346.

Zipes, DP,Wellens, HJ. (1998). Sudden cardiac death. *Circulation,* Vol. 98, No. 21, pp. 2334-2351.

6

Prevention of Sudden Death – Implantable Cardioverter Defibrillator and/or Ventricular Radiofrequency Ablation

Andrea Colella[1], Marzia Giaccardi[2], Antonella Sabatini[3], Alfredo Zuppiroli[2] and Gian Franco Gensini[1]
[1]*Heart and Vessels Department AOU Careggi, Florence*
[2]*Cardiology Department ASL 10, Florence*
[3]*MIT (USA), Finbest, Florence*
[1,2,3]*Italy*
[3]*USA*

1. Introduction

Sudden cardiac death (SCD) is defined as death from cardiac causes occurring unexpectedly within 1 hour of onset of symptoms. About 80% of SCDs are due to ventricular tachyarrhythmia that is, ventricular tachycardia and ventricular fibrillation. The remaining 20% consists of a number of conditions, including cardiomyopathies (10–15%), other structural heart defects (less than 5%) and bradycardia. SCD is responsible for more deaths than cancer, stroke, and AIDS combined (CDC, 2002). The overall incidence of SCD in the United States and Europe is 1 to 2 per 1000 people (0.1% to 0.2%) annually. Almost 80% of all SCDs occur at home. The 10%-25% survival rate is low and has not been improved by the automatic external defibrillator in patients with moderate risk (de Vreede-Swagemakers, 1997; Bardy, 2008; Myerburg, 2001). On the other hand, several clinical trials showed that the implantable cardioverter defibrillator (ICD) could prevent SCD and reduce overall mortality in some patients with severe left ventrocular dysfunction. For these reasons, ICD therapy has become the first choice strategy to prevent SCD from malignant ventricular tachyarrhythmia in high-risk patients. However, there are numerous well-recognized limitations to ICD therapy. These include the effects and the result of appropriate and inappropriate ICD shocks, the cost of the devices, complications related both to the implantation procedure and to subsequent device function, device malfunction, and restricted efficacy despite normal device function in presence of significant concomitant disease and in particular in presence of severe left ventricular disfunction. Several possible solutions have been proposed in the clinical practice, these include better patients' selection for ICD implantation, better ICD programmation, better medical therapy and arrhythmic substrate ablation. The role of catheter ablation of ventricular tachycardia in patients with structural heart disease has been increasing in the last 2 decades. The mechanisms of ventricular tachycardia are now clearer, and the electroanatomic mapping systems have made precise activation and substrate mapping more feasible; therefore, the potential for doing catheter ablation of ventricular tachycardia has increased dramatically in the past several years. Now, multiple and/or unstable ventricular tachycardias, polymorphic ventricular tachycardias, and ventricular fibrillation in selected cases can be targeted by different ablation strategies (Raymond, 2009). General recommendations for the use of catheter ablation are well documented; at this time, an open question remains, namely, whether catheter ablation can replace ICD in patients with structural heart disease.

2. Implantable cardioverter defibrillator

In 1980 Mirowski and colleagues (Mirowski, 1980) implanted the first ICD in a young female with recurrent ventricular fibrillation and provided an innovative approach to aborted SCD. This milestone event started a prolific period of research in SCD prevention and therapy. Although the ICD was considered a treatment of last resort during that incipient stage, subsequent years have witnessed expansion of indications for ICD implantation. (Epstein, 2008). Several large-scale clinical trials have demonstred its efficacy for both primary and secondary prevention of SCD in patients with ischemic and nonischemic cardiomyopathy. The advent of transvenous ICD technology and their potential effects in prevention of SCD elicited also several trials to compare the ICD with conventional antiarrhythmic drug therapy alone. In such high-risk patients, ICD therapy has been shown to improve survival rate compared with a neutral or harmful effect of chronic pharmacological therapy (Dimarco, 2003; Reiffel, 2005). In light of these excellent results, the number of ICD implantations has increased significantly in the last decade, with a simultaneous reduction of the use of stand-alone antiarrhythmic drugs for ventricular indications. (Al-Khatib, 2003; Hine, 1989; Zhan, 2008).

2.1 ICD-related complications

Because of the growing number of ICD patients, ICD-related problems are increasingly encountered and patients undergoing one or multiple shocks are today frequently seen in emergency departments, hospital wards, or ICD clinics.

Therefore, personnel working in these environments should have specific knowledge concerning the management of ICD-related problems. Typically, patients who receive ICDs are at high risk for recurrent arrhythmia; hence, most patients receive one or more ICD treatments for spontaneous arrhythmias after implantation (Dimarco, 2003). Despite the technological evolution of ICD systems, more than 20% of shocks are triggered by supraventricular arrhythmia; thus, they are inappropriate (Dorian, 2004; Nanthakumar, 2000; Rosenqvist, 1998).

The most common cause of inappropriate ICD shocks was atrial fibrillation (44%), followed by other supraventricular tachycardias, including sinus tachycardia (36%), and abnormal sensing (20%) (Daubert, 2008). If appropriate ICD shocks save lives, it may emerge that a few inappropriate shocks are a small price to pay (Raitt, 2008). Inappropriate shocks have a downside. There is a growing medical literature on the adverse psychological consequences of ICD shocks, whether appropriate or not. The ICD shocks are perceived as awfully painful. After an ICD shock, the patient may become immobilized, fearing that any movement or activity might activate another shock. Multiple shocks are the most frightening for patients, causing them to wonder if the device is really working or if it might even kill them. Those individuals who experience an ICD shock exhibit higher levels of psychological distress, anxiety, anger, and depression than those who do not. (Ahmad, 2000; Dunbar, 1993; Dougherty, 1995). The ICD shocks lead to greater psychological distress for family members as well (Luderitz, 1994). Anxiety after ICD shocks remains elevated for an unknown amount of time, and then begins to return to normal levels as long as no further shocks take place (Fricchione, 1989). The level of anxiety, depression, and poor quality of life is comparable in incidence to patients resuscitated from cardiac arrest and cardiopulmonary bypass surgery (Bostwick, 2007). In addition, ICD implantation is associated with neuropsychological impairment that significantly affects acute and long-term cognitive function (Hallas, 2010).

2.2 Electrical storm

Another significant problem is the electrical storm, which is defined as having more than three shocks in a 24-hours period, occurring in 10% to 20% of patients during the first 2 years after ICD implantation (Exner, 2001; Dunbar, 1999). An electrical storm establishes an adverse conditioned response including avoidance of activities that may have been associated with the shocks, leading to heightened self-monitoring of bodily functions, increased anxiety, uncertainty, and increased dependence. In some ICD patients, this condition leads to a reactive depression, helplessness, and post-traumatic stress disorder. In addition, an electrical storm is associated with increased mortality (Credner, 1998; Arya, 2006).

2.3 Mortality in patients with ICD

Inappropriate ICD shocks may not only have adverse psychological consequences but also adverse medical consequences, such as a higher mortality than patients who did not suffer inappropriate shocks, with a hazard ratio of 2.29 ($p=0.025$) (Daubert & Zareba, 2008). Similarly, patients with appropriate shocks also had an increased overall mortality with a hazard ratio between 3 and 4. The higher hazard ratio arises in patients who had both appropriate and inappropriate shocks. In a multivariate analysis, predictors of inappropriate shocks included age > 70 years (hazard ratio 1.9, 95% CI 1.3-2.5; $p=0.01$) and history of atrial fibrillation (hazard ratio 2.0, 95% CI 1.5-2.7; $p<0.01$). The occurrence of only one inappropriate shock showed an all-cause mortality hazard ratio of 1.6 (95% CI 1.1-2.3; $p=0.01$), adjusted for history of atrial fibrillation, age, NYHA functional class, renal function, QRS duration, and beta-blockers use. Each additional inappropriate shock corresponded to a hazard ratio of 1.4 (95% CI 1.2-1.7; $p=0.01$), such that the risk was more than triple after a total of five such shocks (Johannes, 2011). It is interesting to investigate the causality between ICD shocks and an increased risk of death. It is especially reasonable to postulate that patients with progressive heart failure, and therefore increased mortality, might be more likely to develop atrial fibrillation and to suffer inappropriate ICD shocks. These same patients may also be more likely to exhibit ventricular tachycardia or ventricular fibrillation induced by progressive congestive heart failure and to undergo appropriate ICD shocks before dying of congestive heart failure. Depending on the ventricular rate and ICD programming, atrial fibrillation and sinus tachycardia can lead to antitachycardia pacing instead of ICD shocks. If rapid atrial fibrillation and sinus tachycardia were markers for increased mortality, then one would expect inappropriate antitachycardia pacing to be associated with increased mortality as well. In contrast to this expectation, in the MADIT II population, although both appropriate and inappropriate shocks were associated with an increased total mortality, appropriate and inappropriate antitachycardia pacing was not. In fact, having only antitachycardia pacing episodes and no shocks was associated with a trend toward lower mortality. Various likely contributions of ICD shocks to increased total mortality might subsist. Several possible explanations are debated. The first explanation is a direct damage on the myocardium. Animal models have demonstrated a vast array of potentially deleterious effects of DC shocks including alterations in cellular morphology, biochemical function, electrophysiologic function, and hemodynamic function (Tedeschi, 1954; Van Vleet, 1977; Babbs, 1980; Jones, 1980; Wilson, 1988; Trouton, 1992).

Many of the morphologic, biochemical, electrophysiologic and hemodynamic adverse effects of high-intensity DC shocks reported in animals models have also been noted, although with lower frequency, in patients who have received DC shocks of clinically significant intensities. As in animal models, many of these functional changes have been demonstrated to last for minutes to hours as opposed to seconds. The immediacy of post-shock electromechanical dissociation suggests that necrosis is not the cause of the phenomenon. Instead, it is likely that an instantaneous functional abnormality is accountable for electromechanical dissociation. This probability is supported by reports of severe hemodynamic deterioration after internal DC shocks during ICD implantation procedures (Avitall, 1990; Steinbeck, 1994). A severe manifestation of this phenomenon could be expressed as sudden death due to electromechanical dissociation that is the most common mechanism of sudden death in patients with a functioning ICD in place and is associated with high-energy shocks in patients with advanced congestive heart failure. (Mitchell, 2002). The protection afforded by the ICD against sudden arrhythmic death is not absolute, being the rate of sudden death among patients with ICD approximately 5%. If the majority of patients receiving ICDs is similar to those patients included in randomized clinical trials, then ICDs can be expected to be 60 to 70% effective in reducing SCD. This may be more effective than any other available therapy and is thought to be additive to reduction of SCD due to other therapies such as beta-blockers and angiotensin converting enzyme inhibitors. On the other hand, it should serve as a reminder to physicians of the importance of optimization of ICD programming and medical therapy and to patients with regard to compliance with medications and recommended life-style modifications as these measures will reduce their risk (Anderson, 2005).

The second explanation is a possible non-direct damage on the myocardium for the adverse effects of ICD shocks that could direct to increased mortality. We have already outlined the adverse psychological effects of ICD shocks, anxiety and depression, that can set off a cascade of events, including poor compliance to medical therapy, that culminates in an increased risk of death in patients with congestive heart failure. Whether or not there is a causal relationship between ICD shocks and the associated increase in mortality, the psychological effects of shocks alone are reason to do everything possible to reduce the incidence of appropriate and inappropriate shocks (Raitt, 2008).

The extensive implementation of ICD therapy has changed the natural history of ventricular tachycardia (Mason, 1993; Connolly, 2000; AVID Investigators, 1997).

2.4 Approaches to reduce ICD therapy

CDs effectively terminate ventricular arrhythmias through either antitachycardia pacing or shocks and comprise the standard of care for patients at high risk for ventricular arrhythmias. However, ICDs do not prevent the occurrence of ventricular arrhythmias. Patients who, formerly, would have suffered sudden death, now survive to experience recurrent ventricular tachycardia and ICD therapy; thus, shock delivery is administered in a large proportion to patients who have experienced at least one ventricular arrhythmia (Connolly, 2006; Credner, 1998).

2.4.1 Patients selection

There are different approaches to reduce the incidence of appropriate and inappropriate shocks. The first line of defense is good patients' selection for ICD implantation. There is a well-documented increased complication rate for non-guideline-based ICD implantation. In particular, there was an excess of 4 deaths per 1000 ICD implants when the device was implanted outside the guidelines. (Kadish, 2011). The age at implant of patients is very important. Indeed in elderly patients, pooled analysis of the 3 trials considered most relevant to current use of ICDs for primary prevention (MADIT-II, DEFINITE, and SCD-HeFT) showed that prophylactic ICD therapy was associated with a nonsignificant reduction in all-cause mortality compared with medical therapy (HR, 0.81 [95% CI, 0.62 to 1.05]; *P* =0.11). Analyses that included the 2 studies of early enrolled post-acute myocardial infarction patients (DINAMIT and IRIS), also showed no statistically significant decrease in mortality with prophylactic ICD therapy (HR, 0.97 [CI, 0.78 to 1.19]; *P*=0.75) (Santangeli, 2010). Patients who received a non–evidence-based ICD had significantly more comorbidities than patients who received an evidence-based device and were at a higher risk of postprocedural complications (including death). The increased prevalence of comorbidities in recipients of non–evidence based ICDs is unquestionably associated with an increased risk of competing causes of death (Al-Khatib, 2011). While a small risk of complications is acceptable when a procedure has been shown to improve outcomes, no risk is acceptable if a procedure has no demonstrated benefit.

2.4.2 ICD programmation

The second line of defense is ICD programming. In the MADIT II trial, AF was the most common cause of inappropriate shocks. The patients provided with the stability detection algorithm programmed on in their ICDs, which is designed to prevent shocks for atrial fibrillation, were less likely to have inappropriate shocks (Daubert, 2008). Other detection algorithms are available on many ICDs that evaluate the morphology of tachycardias or the timing and frequency of atrial and ventricular activation. They prevent inappropriate shocks for supraventricular rhythms such as atrial fibrillation and sinus tachycardia. These algorithms help to prevent inappropriate shocks. The next step in reducing ICD shocks is programming the devices to use antitachycardia pacing instead of shocks whenever possible. Currently, many electrophysiologists do not routinely program antitachycardia pacing in patients with ICDs. By protocol, antitachycardia pacing was not enabled in the SCD-HeFT (Bardy, 2005). Arguing in favor of the usefulness and efficacy of antitachycardia pacing is the Pain Free II study, which showed that aggressive use of antitachycardia pacing, even for very fast episodes of ventricular tachycardia, was effective and reduced the risk of shocks (Wathen, 2004). Some physicians are concerned that an ineffective antitachycardia pacing will delay tachycardia termination. In response to this concern, one ICD manufacturer has introduced a characteristic in which antitachycardia pacing is used to try to terminate ventricular arrhythmias while the capacitor is charging in preparation for an ICD shock. If the antitachycardia pacing works, the shock is aborted; otherwise, the shock delivery is not delayed. Given the adverse psychological effects of ICD shocks and the possibility that shocks may increase mortality, these programming features should probably be used whenever possible (Raitt, 2008).

2.4.3 Medical therapy

It is less clear whether medical therapy can reduce the risk of ICD shocks. If, in fact, exacerbation of congestive heart failure leads to ICD shocks, perhaps, more aggressive congestive heart failure treatment in patients with ICDs, and use of congestive heart failure monitoring protocols built into some ICDs might prevent some appropriate and inappropriate shocks. It is less clear whether empiric antiarrhythmic therapy prevents ICD shocks; in addition, such therapy cannot be recommended at this time because of the risk of proarrhythmia and the cardiac and noncardiac side effects of antiarrhythmic medications (Raitt, 2008). Beyond aggressive treatment of ischemia and heart failure, preventive treatments for inhibition of ventricular tachycardia are limited. Three agents have been demonstrated in randomized clinical trials to reduce ICD therapies. Amiodarone resulted in a substantial decline in ICD shocks compared with beta-blockers in patients who had experienced prior ventricular arrhythmias. Sotalol moderately reduced shocks (after a 3-week blanking period) in the same population and increased shock-free survival in a placebo-controlled trial (Raitt, 2008). Azimilide has been found to reduce all-cause shocks and symptomatic ventricular tachycardia in a placebo-controlled study (Dorian, 2004). Unfortunately, each of these agents carries significant risk of harmful side-effects. The proarrhythmic mortality risk of sotalol (Waldo, 1996) may be both attenuated in ICD patients, and may be increased in presence of heart failure, diuretic use and older age - all common features of patients with ischemic cardiomyopathy and ventricular tachycardia. Amiodarone use is also associated with a high incidence of adverse effects (Brendorp, 2002), which are moderate at low doses (Vorperian, 1997); on the other hand, they increase with dose and duration such that, in long-term use, side-effects or recurrent arrhythmia are seen very frequently (Bokhari, 2004). Amiodarone use, nephropathy, low left ventricular ejection fraction, and supraventricular tachycardia are independent predictors of cardiac death (Worck, 2007). One can speculate that proarrhythmia and/or increased defibrillation thresholds could play a role in the association with increased mortality (Khalighi, 1997; Zhou, 1998). In addition, amiodarone harmfully affected survival in NYHA III patients in the SCD-HeFT (Bardy, 2005). Azimilide has not demonstrated a change in mortality and is associated with a relatively low rate of torsades de pointes (Camm, 2004; Pratt, 2006), but has not been made available for clinical use. Dronedarone has been associated with higher mortality in the situation of heart failure. Other antiarrhythmic drugs, including dronedarone and dofetilide, have been disappointing, hence, nonpharmacologic alternatives are needed. (Echt, 1991; The CAST Investigators, 1989; DIAMOND studies, 1997; Torp-Pedersen, 1999; Kober, 2008). A good therapeutic alternative to reduce risk of ICD shocks is catheter ablation of ventricular tachycardias.

3. Catheter ablation

In 1987, catheter ablation of ventricular tachycardia was a newly emerging field. The primary therapy for drug refractory ventricular tachycardia was surgical ablation, which was successful in controlling this arrhythmia in 80% to 90% of selected patients, but yielded an operative mortality of 5% to 15% (Cox, 1989). Over the subsequent two decades, significant developments in ablation and mapping technology contributed to improved outcomes: catheter ablation, first, using direct-current energy and radiofrequency current, later. The initial acute success rates using radiofrequency current were on average 75%, with a recurrence rate of 21% over a follow-up time average of 21 months (Gu¨rsoy, 1993; Stevenson, 1993; Gonska, 1994; Kim, 1994; Wilber, 1995; Stevenson, 1998). The limitation of catheter ablation at this time was 2-fold. First, only conventional radiofrequency current (non-irrigated) was available; secondly, only patients with hemodynamically tolerated and stable ventricular tachycardia could be treated, for which an ECG of the spontaneous ventricular tachycardia had been obtained and mapping could be performed during such event (Bogun, 2006; de Chillou, 2002).

3.1 Electroanatomic systems and substrate mapping

The introduction of the electroanatomic mapping system allowed creation of ventricular geometry and displayed low-voltage areas of scar or infarction (Marchlinski, 2000). Mapping during stable sinus or paced rhythm to identify targets for ventricular tachycardia, the so-called substrate mapping (Reddy, 2003; Volkmer, 2006), allows performing catheter ablation in patients with unstable, hemodynamically nontolerated ventricular tachycardia, in patients with multiple ventricular tachycardias, or in patients without inducible ventricular tachycardia (Figure 1).

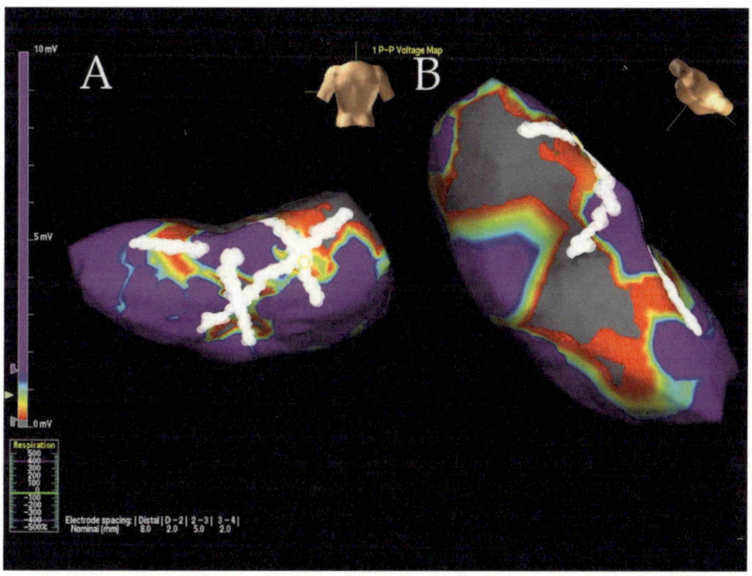

Fig. 1. A and B show the substrate respectively, in the posterior and inferior view in a patient with ischemic dilated cardiomiopathy. In substrate mapping the scar region (grey area) was defined as areas with bipolar local electrogram ≤0.5 mV and the normal myocardium (purple area) was defined as areas with a bipolar local electrogram ≥1.5 mV. The white dots represent the ablation lesions.

Today, most patients with recurrent ventricular tachycardia have an ICD that promptly terminates ventricular tachycardia, so its hemodynamic impact and ECG morphology are often unknown. Thus, substrate mapping is often the only method to perform catheter ablation in patients with an ICD (Kuck, 2009). By selecting catheter ablation for an individual patient, risks and benefits that are determined by patient characteristics, as well as the availability of appropriate facilities with technical expertise should be considered. In the past, catheter ablation of ventricular tachycardia has often been considered a procedure of last resort; now, a recent consensus document has suggested that catheter ablation should generally be considered early in the treatment of patients with recurrent ventricular tachycardia, recognizing that ventricular tachycardia was based mostly upon uncontrolled cohort studies and single-center reports. In the setting of high-risk patients with ICDs, catheter ablation of ventricular tachycardia has been proven to decrease the number of shocks.

3.1.1 Catheter ablation in ischemic patients

In most studies, catheter ablation has been performed in patients with ischemic heart disease after multiple ICD interventions, including patients with incessant ventricular tachycardia. In almost all of these studies, patients were included after failure of 1 or multiple antiarrhythmic drugs. The second largest prospective multicenter trials conducted in the United States using irrigated radiofrequency current included more than 350 patients with structural heart disease, predominantly coronary artery disease (Calkins, 2000; Stevenson, 2008). Both studies differ with respect to patient inclusion and to electrophysiological end-points, but the results were similar. In the cooled radiofrequency current trial, the acute success rate was 71% when the end-point was the elimination of all mappable ventricular tachycardias and 41% when the end-point was the elimination of ventricular tachycardia of any kind. In the thermocool trial, the acute success rate was 49% when elimination of all inducible ventricular tachycardia was used as the end-point. The Kaplan–Meier recurrence rate of sustained ventricular arrhythmia was 56% during 1 year of follow-up. The thermocool trial limited the follow-up time to 6 months for the efficacy end-point. Independence from ventricular tachycardia was 53%. In the thermocool trial, the frequency of ventricular tachycardia was reduced by ≥75% in 67% of patients. An increase in the number of ventricular tachycardia episodes was observed in 20% of patients. Patients with ventricular tachycardia recurrences were older, had more heart failure, more atrial fibrillation, multiple myocardial infarction sites, and more inducible ventricular tachycardias; they received more radiofrequency lesions, and more often, had a ventricular tachycardia inducible after ablation compared with patients without ventricular tachycardia recurrences. In the cooled radiofrequency current study, a ≥75% reduction in the ventricular tachycardia frequency in the two months after ablation compared to the two months before ablation was observed in 99 of 122 patients (81%), of whom 115 had an ICD. Only the absence of an inducible ventricular tachycardia, recognized as the clinical ventricular tachycardia, was a predictor of clinical success. Another European multicenter study (Euro-VT study) performed catheter ablation using external irrigation in 63 patients with recurrent scar-related ventricular tachycardia (Tanner, 2009). Catheter ablation was acutely successful in 51 patients (81%). During a mean follow-up of 12 ± 3 months, 31 patients (49%, 19 of 51 initially successfully ablated patients and 12 of 12 unsuccessfully ablated patients) experienced ventricular tachycardia recurrence. However, even among the patients with recurrence, the number of ICD therapies was significantly reduced in 79% of the cases. One limitation of catheter ablation studies in ICD patients must be addressed. In almost all studies, antiarrhythmic drugs were not systematically withdrawn after ablation. Therefore, any beneficial effect of catheter ablation in these studies may be influenced by drug therapy, even when most patients were drug failures before ventricular tachycardia ablation. While the above-mentioned and previously conducted studies clearly showed the beneficial effect of catheter ablation of ventricular tachycardia with respect to ventricular tachycardia recurrence, the periprocedural mortality should also be considered in these patients. Indeed, the effectiveness of catheter ablation in ICD patients must be balanced with the safety profile of this interventional procedure. The reported procedure-related mortality ranges from 0% to 3.5%. In addition, major complications including stroke, myocardial infarction, tamponade, valve injury, and atrio-ventricular block occurred in 8-10% of the patients. In the Euro-VT study, the rate of major complications was only 1.6% and the 1-year mortality in these studies reached 8-18%.

3.1.2 Catheter ablation in nonischemic patients

Data on catheter ablation in ICD patients with nonischemic ventricular tachycardia from large multicenter trials are lacking. The anatomic substrate is different in patients with nonischemic ventricular tachycardia, since more extensive scar is often present in the epicardium and not in the endocardium, compared with the majority of patients with a previous myocardial infarct. In both groups, epicardial ablation has been successfully applied after failure of endocardial ablation. In general, acute success rates of catheter ablation are similar to ischemic ventricular tachycardia patients, but recurrence rates seem to be higher (Soejima, 2004; Delacretaz, 2000; Nazarian, 2005; Verma, 2005; Dalal, 2007). Moreover, catheter ablation has been shown to eliminate electrical storm in patients with and without underlying heart disease by either inhibiting the trigger factors for ventricular tachycardia/ventricular fibrillation, namely ventricular premature beats, or by modifying the substrate for ventricular tachycardia/ventricular fibrillation. Catheter ablation significantly reduces the number of ICD interventions in patients with electrical storm (Della Bella, 2004). In a recent single-center study, 95 patients with electrical storm, leading to a mean number of 14 ICD shocks per patient per day, underwent catheter ablation. Seventy-two patients had underlying coronary artery disease, 10 patients had dilated cardiomyopathy, and 13 patients had right ventricular disease. After catheter ablation, electrical storm was acutely suppressed in all patients and did not recur during follow-up of 22 months in patients in whom either no ventricular tachycardia could be induced or clinical ventricular tachycardia became noninducible. Furthermore, death from any cause could significantly be reduced in both groups compared with patients in whom the clinical ventricular tachycardia remained inducible and electrical storm recurred. Both cardiac death as well as sudden cardiac death was significantly higher in patients with electrical storm recurrences (50% versus 0%). This observation indicates that a successful ventricular tachycardia ablation procedure may be associated with a reduction of total mortality in subgroups of patients. The procedure typically is prompted by frequent defibrillator therapies despite multiple combinations of antiarrhythmic drugs. Use of catheter ablation earlier during the clinical course of ventricular tachycardia, soon after its onset, may be beneficial.

3.1.3 Prophylactic catheter ablation

The role of prophylactic radiofrequency catheter ablation of arrhythmogenic substrate in patients with a previous myocardial infarction in preventing ICD therapy was evaluated in the Substrate Mapping and Ablation in Sinus Rhythm to Halt Ventricular Tachycardia (SMASH-VT) trial and in the Catheter ablation of stable ventricular tachycardia before defibrillator implantation in patients with coronary heart disease (VTACH) trial (Reddy,

2007; Kuck, 2010). SMASH-VT was a prospective randomized three-center trial of catheter ablation versus no intervention for patients with implantation of a secondary prophylactic ICD within the prior 6 months or who had received recent appropriate ICD therapy. Catheter ablation resulted in reduced appropriate ICD therapy from 33 to 12% (hazard ratio 0.35). Secondary end-points included a reduction in ventricular tachycardia storm, but no effect on total mortality occurred. Although this landmark study demonstrated proof of the principle that catheter ablation can have a favorable effect, limitations such as the lack of adjudicator blinding, stratification and standard ICD programming make the results more difficult to interpret. Most importantly, the role of antiarrhythmic drugs was not addressed by this study design, limiting direct applicability of the results to clinical practice (El-Damaty, & Sapp, 2011). VTACH trial was similar in design to that of SMASH-VT. One hundred and ten patients presenting with ventricular tachycardia and prior myocardial infarction were randomly allocated to catheter ablation or no intervention, followed by ICD implantation. Antiarrhythmic drug use was discouraged, and not significantly different between groups. Patients were stratified by center and ejection fraction (cut-off 30%); a blinded committee adjudicated outcomes and ICD programming was standardized. The VTACH trial showed that catheter ablation, performed before ICD implantation in patients after the first episode of a hemodynamically stable ventricular tachycardia, significantly prolonged the median time to first ventricular tachycardia/ventricular fibrillation from 5.9 months to 18.6 months. The benefit was more pronounced in patients with left ventricular ejection fraction > 30% (Figure 2).

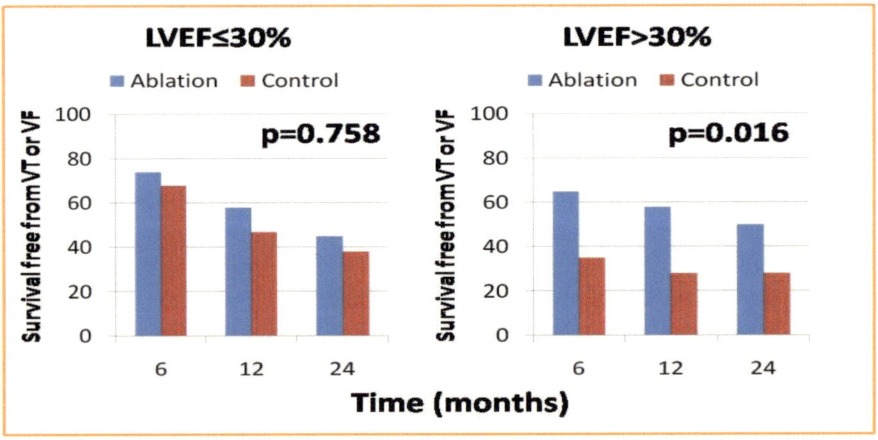

Modified from Kuck et al., Lancet, 2010

Fig. 2. Survival free from ventricular tachycardia (VT) or ventricular fibrillation (VF) in patients with left-ventricular ejection fraction (LVEF) less or equal than 30% and left-ventricular ejection fraction greater than 30%.

Furthermore, catheter ablation reduced the overall incidence of appropriate ICD interventions by 28% and the incidence of ICD shocks by 43%. Even more importantly, catheter ablation reduced the median number of appropriate ICD interventions per patient and year of follow-up by 93%. In addition, catheter ablation significantly reduced the rate of hospitalizations for cardiac reasons. This well designed trial provides further support for the effectiveness of catheter ablation in reducing ventricular tachycardia events, but does not give clinical guidance on the relative role of catheter ablation in comparison to antiarrhythmic drug therapy. The complication rate becomes even more important if an interventional procedure is performed prophylactically. In both trials, the incidence of ablation related death was 0% and of major complications 4.7% and 3.8%, respectively. The event rate in the control group of the VTACH trial was roughly twice as that observed in SMASH-VT, but the relative reduction in events was similar, at 35–40%.

3.2 Open questions in VT catheter ablation

3.2.1 The role of antiarrhythmic therapy

Many important questions remain. Should ablation be preferred over antiarrhythmic drugs? The largest prospective, randomized trial evaluating several drug regimen in patients with an ICD for secondary prevention showed that the combination of beta-blockers and amiodarone had the greatest effect, with a reduction of ICD shocks by 73% compared to the control group (beta-blocker alone) and of 57% compared to the sotalol group, with an incidence of ICD shocks in the control group of approximately 30% after 1 year (Connolly, SJ et al. 2006). In a previous trial, sotalol reduced the risk of death from any cause or the delivery of a first shock for any reason by 48%. Furthermore, sotalol reduced the probability of the delivery of an appropriate first ICD shock or a first shock of any reason (Pacifico, 1999). Sotalol also prevented the occurrence of shocks in response to supraventricular arrhythmias, a frequent cause of inappropriate defibrillator therapy. Despite these beneficial effects, drug efficacy depends on patient compliance. In particular, if a lifetime therapy is required and is associated with side effects, this may lead to a discontinuation of drugs therapy. Furthermore, antiarrhythmic drugs such as amiodarone may increase the defibrillation threshold (Hohnloser, 2006). Even if this may not play a significant role in the majority of patients with modern devices, it can be harmful in the individual patient. In a randomized clinical trial comparing cooled radiofrequency catheter ablation of ventricular tachycardia and drugs therapy, arrhythmic recurrences was significantly lower with cooled ablation than with drug therapy. (Epstein, 1998).

Regarding catheter ablation procedural outcomes, multiple small series, single center of catheter ablation for ventricular tachycardia have reported freedom from recurrent ventricular tachycardia in 50-80% of patients over follow-up, which ranges from 6 to 18 months. Long-term results are sparse, and completeness of reported follow-ups is sometimes suboptimal. Patients remained on antiarrhythmic drugs (amiodarone 94% and sotalol 5%) postprocedure and those with persistently inducible clinical ventricular tachycardia had shorter time to death, and shorter time to ventricular tachycardia recurrence and were the only patients with recurrence of ventricular tachycardia storm (Carbucicchio, 2008).

3.2.2 The role of ventricular function

In our experience, among the 66 patients referred to our clinic for radiofrequency catheter ablation of recurrent post infarction ventricular tachycardias, only 19 (29%) showed recurrences during a mean follow-up of 26 ± 12 months. This finding "per se" highlights the role of radiofrequency catheter ablation in the overall clinical management of recurrent post infarction ventricular tachycardias in patients with ICD. In addition, our findings stressed the role of poor left ventricular function as an independent predictor of recurrent ventricular tachycardia. Among patients with ejection fraction < 35%, 11 out of 25 (44%) still continued to have ventricular tachycardia recurrences, independently of whether the ventricular tachycardia responsible for ICD therapies was inducible at the end of the procedure or not. Most clinical trials (Moss, 2004; Moss, 1996; Buxton, 1999; Bardy, 2005) testing the efficacy of antiarrhythmic versus ICD therapy have used the ejection fraction as the marker for advanced disease, with the qualifying criteria in the range of 30–40% or less. Interestingly, in the AVID trial (Domanski, 1999) a subgroup analysis suggested that there was no benefit of ICD therapy over amiodarone for patients with ejection fraction between 36% and 40%, being all the benefit accrued to those patients with ejection fraction 35% or less. This observation raises the critical question we addressed in conceiving this study, about predictors of ventricular tachycardia recurrences, and consequently about therapeutic options, for patients with ejection fraction greater than 35%. Our findings show that, among patients with ejection fraction >35% and <50%, no recurrent ventricular tachycardia was further detected in the patients in whom the ventricular tachycardia responsible for ICD therapies was not inducible at the end of the procedure (100% specificity). Whereas ventricular tachycardia recurrences continued only in the patients, in whom the clinical ventricular tachycardia was inducible (100% sensitivity) (Colella, 2009). Actually, inducibility of the clinical ventricular tachycardia, more than being a predictor of ventricular tachycardia recurrences, is simply the consequence of radiofrequency catheter ablation failure (Della Bella, 2002), i.e. of the fact that the clinical ventricular tachycardia has not been successfully ablated. Accordingly, at least in patients with ejection fraction >35% and <50%, the procedure should be repeated until an acutely successful ablation of the clinical ventricular tachycardia is achieved. For these patients, indeed, radiofrequency catheter ablation might be considered a reasonable alternative to ICD as the first choice. Finally, our findings show that in all the 24 patients with ejection fraction >50% no recurrent ventricular tachycardia was any longer detected during the follow-up. Based upon our findings, a simple algorithm (Figure 3) is proposed for the management of recurrent ventricular

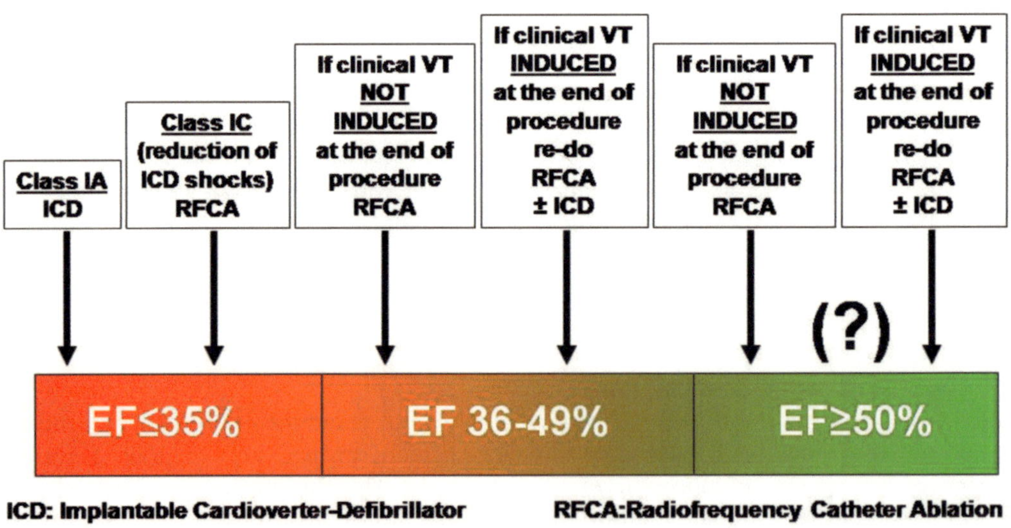

Fig. 3. Algorithm for the management of recurrent Ventricular Tachycardias in patients with previous Myocardial Infarction.

tachycardias in patients with previous myocardial infarction: a) for patients with ejection fraction ≤35%, ICD still remains the first choice (class 1A). However, radiofrequency catheter ablation is indicated to reduce ICD shocks (class 1C) (Zipes, 2006), b) for patients with ejection fraction >35% and <50%, the first choice might be radiofrequency catheter ablation and any effort should be made to successfully ablate the VT, repeating the procedure if needed. The implantation of ICD might be limited to those patients in whom the ventricular tachycardia is not successfully ablated. c) For patients with EF ≥50%, the first choice might be radiofrequency catheter ablation.

4. Conclusions

In conclusion, the published studies have shown the important role of catheter ablation in patients with structural heart disease and ICD implantation who experienced appropriate ICD therapy due to recurrent ventricular tachycardias. Successful catheter ablation in these patients prevents or reduces the number of ventricular tachycardia recurrences as well as the rate of ICD shocks, improving the quality of life and probably long-term mortality.

Finally, the question whether ablation can replace ICD in patients with structural heart disease is presented. The results of recently published studies are promising for further expansion of ventricular tachycardia ablation indication, but several points merit additional consideration. Catheter ablation of ventricular tachycardia is still an extremely complex procedure and the reported results reflect the outcome of such ablations from highly experienced and high-volume centers and, therefore, cannot be extrapolated to all electrophysiology departments without additional simplification and standardization of the ablation procedures and strategies. In spite of being able to achieve acute complete success in the majority of patients who underwent catheter ablation of ventricular tachycardia, accurate long-term prediction of outcome based on current risk predictors is difficult. Therefore, we cannot currently replace ICD with catheter ablation, although in selected patients, with hemodynamically stable and/or slow ventricular tachycardia and preserved or mildly reduced left ventricular function (for which data from randomized studies are lacking), catheter ablation might be considered an alternative to ICD. In addition, even upon developing more effective ablation strategies and finding good predictors of long-term outcome after a single center ablation procedure, the substrate of arrhythmia in patients with structural heart disease is dynamic. Due to this inherently dynamic characteristics of the arrhythmic substrate, cardioverter defibrillator implantation, cannot be replaced in the long-term, with catheter ablation of ventricular tachycardia. It is in fact necessary to stratify the risk repetitively and regularly, in order to perform repeated ablation procedures, if necessary. Thus, before widespread recommendation of catheter ablation of ventricular tachycardia becomes evident, especially prophylactic ablation, standardizing the ablation procedure and strategies, endpoints, and the follow-up should be performed. Further studies are necessary to clarify the role of catheter ablation of ventricular tachycardia on long-term mortality of patients with structural heart disease (Arya, 2009). ICD remains a life-saving device for patients with sustained ventricular tachycardia late after myocardial infarction; but in selected patients, especially in patients with ejection fraction > 30%, who are receiving an ICD for stable ventricular tachycardia, arrhythmic substrate ablation can be considered early. Evidence of a positive effect on survival, subsequent hospital admissions, or quality of life is needed before catheter ablation can be recommended for routine use. We believe that today's trial is further evidence to support early use of catheter ablation, as a valid alternative to antiarrhythmic drug therapy, for symptomatic recurrent ventricular tachycardia after ICD implantation, provided that expertise to safely perform the procedure is available (Stevenson, 2010).

5. References

Ahmad, M; Bloomstein, L; Roelke, M; Bernstein, AD; Parsonnet, V. Patients' attitudes toward implanted defibrillator shocks. *Pacing Clin Electrophysiol*, Vol. 23, (2000), pp. 934–8, ISSN 1540-8159

Aliot, EM; Stevenson, WG; Almendral–Garrote, JM EHRA/HRS Expert Consensus on Catheter Ablation of Ventricular arrhythmias. *Europace* , Vol. 11:, (2009), pp 771-817, ISSN 1099-5129.

Al-Khatib, SM; LaPointe, NM; Curtis, LH; Kramer, JM; Swann, J; Honig, P; Califf, RM. Outpatient prescribing of antiarrhythmic drugs from 1995 to 2000. *Am J Cardiol*, Vol. 91, (2003), pp 91–94, ISSN 1076-7460

Al-Khatib, SM; Hellkamp, A; Curtis, J; Mark, D; Peterson, E; Sanders, GD; Heidrenreich, PA; Hernandez, AF; Curtis, LH; Hammill, S. Non-Evidence-Based ICD Implantation in the United States. *JAMA*, Vol. 305, (2011), pp 43-49, ISSN 1538-3598

Anderson, KP. Sudden Cardiac Death Unresponsive to Implantable Defibrillator Therapy: An Urgent Target for Clinicians, Industry and Government. *Journal of Interventional Cardiac Electrophysiology*, Vol, 14, (2005), pp 71-78, ISSN 1532-2092

Arya, A; Haghjoo, M; Dehghani, MR. Prevalence and predictors of electrical storm in patients with implantable cardioverter-defibrillator. *Am J Cardiol*, Vol. 97, (2006), pp 389-392, ISSN 1076-7460

Arya, A; Piorkowski, C; Kircher, S; Sommer, P; Bollmann, A; Gaspar, T; Hindricks, G. Results of recent Studies in Catheter Ablation of Ventricular tachycardias. In Whom to Abandon the ICD? *Herz*, Vol. 34, (2009), pp 539-544.

AVID Investigators. The Antiarrhythmics versus Implantable Defibrillators Investigators. A comparison of antiarrhythmic-drug therapy with implantable defibrillators in patients resuscitated from near-fatal ventricular arrhythmias. *N Engl J Med*, Vol. 337, (1997), pp. 1576–1583, ISSN 1533-4406

Avitall, B; Port, S; Gal, R. Automatic implantable cardioverter/defibrillator discharges and acute myocardial injury. *Circulation*, Vol. 81, (1990), pp 1482–1487, ISSN 1524-4539

Babbs, CF; Tacker, WA; Van Vleet, JF; Bourland, JD; Geddes, LA. Therapeutic indices for transchest defibrillator shocks: effective, damaging, and lethal electrical doses. *Am Heart J*, Vol. 99, (1980), pp 734–8, ISSN 1097-6744

Bardy, GH; Lee, KL; Mark, DB et al., Sudden Cardiac Death in Heart Failure Trial (SCD-HeFT) Investigators. Amiodarone or an implantable cardioverter-defibrillator for congestive heart failure. *N Engl J Med*, Vol. 352, (2005), 225–37, ISSN 1533-4406

Bardy, GH; Lee, KL; Mark, DB; et al. HAT Investigators. Home use of automated external defibrillators for sudden cardiac arrest. *N Engl J Med*, Vol. 358, (2008), pp 1793–1804 ISSN 1533-4406

Bogun, F; Kim, HM; Han, J; et al. Comparison of mapping criteria for hemodynamically tolerated, postinfarction ventricular tachycardia. *Heart Rhythm* Vol. 3, (2006), pp 20 –26 ISSN 1547-5271

Bokhari, F; Newman, D; Greene, M et al. Long-term comparison of the implantable cardioverter defibrillator versus amiodarone: eleven-year followup of a subset of patients in the Canadian Implantable Defibrillator Study (CIDS). *Circulation* Vol. 110, (2004), pp 112–116, ISSN 1524-4539

Bostwick, JM & Sola, CL. An updated review of implantable cardioverter/defibrillators, induced anxiety, and quality of life. *Psychiatr Clin North Am.* Vol. 30, (2007), pp 677–688, ISSN 0193-953X

Brendorp, B; Pedersen, O; Torp-Pedersen, C et al. A benefit-risk assessment of class III antiarrhythmic agents. *Drug Saf* Vol. 25, (2002), pp 847–865, ISSN 0114-5916

Buxton, AE; Lee, KL; Fisher, JD; et al. A randomized study of the prevention of sudden death in patients with coronary artery disease. *N Eng J Med,* Vol. 341, (1999), pp1882–1890, ISSN 1533-4406

Calkins, H; Epstein, A; Packer, et al. Catheter ablation of ventricular tachycardia in patients with structural heart disease using cooled radiofrequency energy: results of a prospective multicenter study. *JACC,* Vol. 35, (2000), pp 1905–1914, ISSN 1558-3597

Camm, AJ; Pratt, CM; Schwartz, PJ.Mortality in patients after a recent myocardial infarction: a randomized, placebo-controlled trial of azimilide using heart rate variability for risk stratification. *Circulation,* Vol. 109, (2004), pp 990–996, ISSN 1524-4539

Carbucicchio, C; Santamaria, M; Trevisi, N et al. Catheter ablation for the treatment of electrical storm in patients with implantable cardioverter-defibrillators. Short- and long-term outcomes in a prospective single-center study. *Circulation* , Vol. 117, (2008), pp 462–469, ISSN 1524-4539.

Cardiac Arrhythmia Suppression Trial (CAST) Investigators. Preliminary report: effect of encainide and flecainide on mortality in a randomized trial of arrhythmia suppression after myocardial infarction. *N Engl J Med,* Vol. 321, (1989), pp 406–412, ISSN 1533-4406

Centers for Disease Control and Prevention (CDC). State-Specific Mortality from Sudden Cardiac Death-United States,1999. *Morb Mortal Wkly Rep (MMWR),* Vol. 51, (2002), pp 123-126, ISSN 1581-861X

Colella, A; Giaccardi, M; Molino Lova, R; et al. Ventricular tachycardia inducibility after radiofrequency ablation affects the outcomes in patients with coronary artery disease and implantable cardioverter-defibrillators: The role of left ventricular function, *J Interv Card Electrophysiol,* Vol. 25,(2009), pp229–234, ISSN 1572-8595

Connolly, SJ; Dorian, P; Roberts, RS; et al. Optimal Pharmacological Therapy in Cardioverter Defibrillator Patients (OPTIC) Investigators. Comparison of B-blockers, amiodarone plus beta-blockers, or sotalol for prevention of shocks from implantable cardioverter defibrillators: the OPTIC study: a randomized trial. *JAMA,* Vol. 295, (2006), pp 165–171, ISSN 1538-3598

Connolly, SJ; Gent, M; Roberts, RS et al. Canadian implantable defibrillator study (CIDS): a randomized trial of the implantable cardioverter defibrillator against amiodarone. *Circulation,* Vol. 101, (2000), pp 1297–1302, ISSN 1524-4539

Cox, JL. Patient selection criteria and results of surgery for refractory ischemic ventricular tachycardia. *Circulation,* Vol. 79, (1989), pp I163–I177, ISSN 1524-4539

Credner, SC; Klingenheben, T; Mauss, O et al. Electrical storm in patients with transvenous implantable cardioverter-defibrillators: incidence, management and prognostic implications. *JACC*, Vol. 32, (1998), pp 1909–1915, ISSN 1558-3597

Dalal, D; Jain, R; Tandri, H; et al. Long-term efficacy of catheter ablation of ventricular tachycardia in patients with arrhythmogenic right ventricular dysplasia/cardiomyopathy. *JACC*, Vol. 50, (2007), pp 432– 440, ISSN 1558-3597

Daubert, JP; Zareba, W; Cannom, DS et al., for the MADIT II Investigators. Inappropriate implantable cardioverter-defibrillators shocks in the MADIT II study: frequency, mechanisms, predictors, and survival impact. *JACC*, Vol. 51, (2008), pp1357– 65, ISSN 1558-3597

de Chillou, C; Lacroix, D; Klug, D; et al. Isthmus characteristics of reentrant ventricular tachycardia after myocardial infarction. *Circulation*, Vol. 105, (2002), pp726–731., ISSN 1524-4539

de Vreede-Swagemakers, JJ; Gorgels, AP; Dubois-Arbouw, WI; et al. Out-of-hospital cardiac arrest in the 1990s: a population-based study in the Maastricht area on incidence, characteristics and survival. *JACC*, Vol. 30, (1997), pp1500–1505, ISSN 1558-3597

Delacretaz, E; Stevenson, WG; Ellison, KE; et al. Mapping and radiofrequency catheter ablation of the three types of sustained monomorphic ventricular tachycardia in nonischemic heart disease. *J Cardiovasc Electrophysiol*, Vol. 11, (2000), pp11–17, ISSN 1532-2092

Della Bella, P; Riva, S; Fassini, G; et al. Incidence and significance of pleomorphism in patients with postmyocardial infarction ventricular tachycardia: acute and long-term outcome of radiofrequency catheter ablation. *Eur Heart J*, Vol. 25, (2004), pp1127–1138, ISSN 1522-9645

Della Bella, P; De Ponti, R; Uriarte, JA; et al. Catheter ablation and antiarrhythmic drugs for haemodynamically tolerated post-infarction ventricular tachycardia. Long-term outcome in relation to acute electrophysiological findings. *Eur Heart J*, Vol. 23, (2002), pp 414–424, ISSN 1522-9645

DIAMOND. Dofetilide in patients with left ventricular dysfunction and either heart failure or acute myocardial infarction: rationale, design, and patient characteristics of the DIAMOND studies. Danish Investigations of Arrhythmia and Mortality ON Dofetilide. *Clin Cardiol Vol.* 20, (1997), pp 704–710, ISSN 0160-9289

Dimarco, JP. Implantable cardioverter-defibrillators. *N Engl J Med*, Vol. 349, (2003), pp1836 – 1847, ISSN 1533-4406

Dofetilide in patients with left ventricular dysfunction and either heart failure or acute myocardial infarction: rationale, design, and patient characteristics of the DIAMOND studies. Danish Investigations of Arrhythmia and Mortality ON Dofetilide. *Clin Cardiol* Vol. 20, (1997), pp 704–710, ISSN 0160-9289

Domanski, MJ; Saksena, S; Epstein, AE; et al. Relative effectiveness of the implantable cardioverter-defibrillator and antiarrhytmic drugs in patients with varying degrees of left ventricular dysfunction who have survived malignant ventricular arrhythmia. AVID investigators. Antiarrhytmic Versus implantable Defibrillators. *JACC*, Vol. 34, (1999), pp 1090–1095, ISSN 1558-3597

Dorian, P; Borggrefe, M; Al-Khalidi, HR et al. Placebo-controlled, randomized clinical trial of azimilide for prevention of ventricular tachyarrhythmias in patients with an implantable cardioverter defibrillator. *Circulation* , Vol. 110, (2004), pp 3646–3654. ISSN 1524-4539

Dorian, P; Philippon, F, Thibault, B; et al. Randomized controlled study of detection enhancements versus rate-only detection to prevent inappropriate therapy in a dual-chamber implantable cardioverter-defibrillator. *Heart Rhythm*, Vol. 1, (2004), pp540 –547, ISSN 1547-5271

Dougherty, CM; Shaver, JF. Psychophysiological responses after sudden cardiac arrest during hospitalization. *Appl Nurs Res*, Vol. 8, (1995), pp160–8, ISSN 1532-8201

Dunbar, SB; Warner, CD; Purcell, JA. Internal cardioverter defibrillator device discharge: experiences of patients and family members. *Heart Lung*, Vol. 22, (1993), pp 494 - 501, ISSN 1547-5271

Dunbar, SB; Kimble, LP; Jenkins, LS et al. Association of mood disturbance and arrhythmia events in patients after cardioverter defibrillator implantation. *Depress Anxiety*, Vol. 9, (1999), pp163– 8, 1520-6394, ISSN 1520-6394

Echt, DS; Liebson, PR; Mitchell, LB et al. Mortality and morbidity in patients receiving encainide, flecainide, or placebo. The Cardiac Arrhythmia Suppression Trial. *N Engl J Med*, Vol. 324, (1991), pp781–788, 1533-4406, ISSN 1533-4406

El-Damaty, A & Sapp JL. The role of catheter ablation for ventricular tachycardia in patients with ischemic heart disease. *Current Opinion in Cardiology*, Vol. 26, (2011), pp30-39, ISSN 0268-4705

Epstein, AE; Wilber, DJ; Wharton, JM; et al. Randomized Controlled Trial of Ventricular tachycardia Treatment by Cooled tip Catheter Ablation vs Drug Therapy. *JACC*, Vol. 1998 Abstract 1046-167, pp 118A, ISSN 1558-3597

Epstein, AE; Di Marco, JP; Ellenbogen, KA; et al. ACC/AHA/HRS 2008 Guidelines for Device-Based Therapy of Cardiac Rhythm Abnormalities: a report of the American College of Cardiology/American Heart Association Task Force on Practice Guidelines (Writing Committee to Revise the ACC/AHA/NASPE 2002 Guideline Update for Implantation of Cardiac Pacemakers and Antiarrhythmia Devices): developed in collaboration with the American Association for Thoracic Surgery and Society of Thoracic Surgeons. *Circulation*, Vol. 117, (2008), pp e350–e408, ISSN 1524-4539

Exner, DV; Pinski, SL; Wyse, DG et al. Electrical storm presages non sudden death: the Antiarrhythmics Versus Implantable Defibrillators (AVID) trial. *Circulation*, Vol.103, (2001), pp 2066 –71, ISSN 1524-4539

Fricchione, GL; Olson, LC; Vlay, SC. Psychiatric syndromes in patients with the automatic internal cardioverter defibrillator: anxiety, psychological dependence, abuse, and withdrawal. *Am Heart J*, Vol. 117, (1998), pp1411–4, ISSN 1097-6744

Gonska, BD; Cao, K; Schaumann, A; et al. Catheter ablation of ventricular tachycardia in 136 patients with coronary artery disease: results and long-term follow-up. *JACC*, Vol. 24, (1994), pp1506 –1514, ISSN 1558-3597

Gu¨rsoy, S; Chiladakis, I; Kuck, KH. First lessons from radiofrequency catheter ablation in patients with ventricular tachycardia. *PACE* Vol. 16, (1993), pp687– 691, ISSN 1540-8159

Hallas, CN; Burke, LJ; White, DG; Connelly, DT. A Prospective 1-Year Study of Changes in Neuropsycological Functioning After Implantable Cardioverter-Defibrillator Surgery. *Circ Arrhythm Electrophysiol* , Vol 3, (2010), pp170-177, ISSN 1941-3149

Hine, LK; Gross, TP; Kennedy, DL. Outpatient antiarrhythmic drug use from 1970 through 1986. *Arch Intern Med.*, Vol. 149, (1989), pp1524 –1527, ISSN 1536-3679

Hohnloser, SH; Dorian, P; Roberts, R; et al. Effect of amiodarone and sotalol on ventricular defibrillation threshold: the optimal pharmacological therapy in cardioverter defibrillator patients (OPTIC) trial. *Circulation*, Vol. 114, (2006), pp 104–109, ISSN 1524-4539

Johannes, B; van Rees, JB; Borleffs, CJW; et al. Inappropriate implantable cardioverter-defibrillator shocks incidence, predictors, and impact on mortality. *JACC*, Vol. 57, (2011), pp 556-562, ISSN 1558-3597

Jones, JL; Paull, WK; Lepeschkin, E; Jones, RE. Ultrastructural injury to chick myocardial cells in vitro following electric countershock. *Circ Res* Vol. 46, (1980), pp 387–94, ISSN 1524-2092

Kadish, A & Goldberger, J. Selecting Patients for ICD implantation. Are Clinicians Choosing Appropriately? *JAMA*, Vol. 305, (2011), pp 91-92, ISSN 1538-3598

Khalighi, MD; Daly, MD; Leino, PEV; et al. Clinical predictors of transvenous defibrillation energy requirements. *Am J Cardiol*, Vol. 79, (1997), pp150–153, ISSN 0002-9149

Kim, YH; Sosa-Suarez, G; Trouton, TG; et al. Treatment of ventricular tachycardia by transcatheter radiofrequency ablation in patients with ischemic heart disease. Circulation, Vol. 89, (1994), pp1094 –1102, ISSN 1524-4539

Kober, L; Torp-Pedersen, C; McMurray, JJ. Increased mortality after dronedarone therapy for severe heart failure. *N Engl J Med*, Vol. 358, (2008), pp 2678–2687, ISSN 1533-4406

Kuck, KH; Should Catheter Ablation be the Preferred Therapy for Reducing ICD Shocks? Ventricular Tachycardia in Patients With an Implantable Defibrillator Warrants Catheter Ablation. Circ Arrhythm Electrophysiol, Vol. 2, (2009), pp713-720, ISSN 1941-3149

Kuck, KH; Schaumann, A; Eckardt, L et al, for the VTACH study group. Catheter ablation of stable ventricular tachycardia before defibrillator implantation in patients with coronary heart disease (VTACH): a multicentre randomised controlled trial. *Lancet*, Vol. 375, (2010), pp31–4, ISSN 1470-2045

Luderitz, B; Jung, W; Deister, A; et al. Patient acceptance of implantable cardioverter defibrillator devices: changing attitudes. Am Heart J, Vol. 127, (1994), pp 1179–84, ISSN 1097-6744

Marchlinski FE, Callans DJ, Gottlieb CD, Zado E. Linear ablation lesions for control of unmappable ventricular tachycardia in patients with ischemic and nonischemic cardiomyopathy. *Circulation*, Vol. 101, (2000), pp1288–1296, ISSN 1524-4539

Mason, JW. A comparison of electrophysiologic testing with Holter monitoring to predict antiarrhythmic-drug efficacy for ventricular tachyarrhythmias. Electrophysiologic

Study versus Electrocardiographic Monitoring Investigators. *N Engl J Med*, Vol. 9, (1993), pp 445–451, ISSN 1533-4406

Mirowski, M; Reid, PR; Mower, MM; et al. Termination of malignant ventricular arrhythmias with an implanted automatic defibrillator in human beings. *N Engl J Med*, Vol. 303, (1980), pp 322–324, ISSN 1533-4406

Mitchell, LB; Pineda, EA; Titus, JL; Bartosch, PM; Benditt, DG. Sudden Death in Patients With Implantable Cardioverter Defibrillators. The Importance of Post-Shock Electromechanical Dissociation. *JACC*, Vol. 39, (2002), pp 1323-1328, ISSN 1558-3597

Morady, F; Harvey, M; Kalbfleisch, SJ; el-Atassi, R; Calkins, H; Langberg, JJ. Radiofrequency catheter ablation of ventricular tachycardia in patients with coronary artery disease. *Circulation*, Vol. 87 (1993), pp 363–372, ISSN 1524-4539.

Moss, AJ; Greenberg, H; Case, RB; Zareba, W; Hall, WJ; Brown, MW et al. Multicenter Automatic Defibrillator Implantation Trial-II Research Group. Long-term clinical course of patients after termination of ventricular tachyarrhythmia by an implanted defibrillator. *Circulation*, Vol. 110, (2004), pp 3760–3765, ISSN 1524-4539.

Moss, AJ., Hall,W. J., Cannom, D. S., Daubert, J. P., Higgins, S. L., Klein, H., et al. Improved survival with an implanted defibrillator in patients with coronary disease al high risk for ventricular arrythmia. *N Engl J Med*, Vol. 335,1, (1996), pp 933–1940, ISSN 1533-4406

Myerburg, RJ. Sudden cardiac death: exploring the limits of our knowledge. *J Cardiovasc Electrophysiol.*, Vol. 12, (2001), pp 369–381, ISSN 1532-2092

Nanthakumar, K; Paquette, M; Newman, D; Deno, DC; Malden, L; Gunderson, B; Gilkerson, J; Greene, M; Heng, D; Dorian P. Inappropriate therapy from atrial fibrillation and sinus tachycardia in automated implantable cardioverter defibrillators. *Am Heart J*, Vol. 139, (2000), 797–803, ISSN 1097-6744

Nazarian, S; Bluemke, DA; Lardo, AC; Zviman, MM; Watkins, SP; Dickfeld, TL; Meininger, GR; Roguin, A; Calkins, H; Tomaselli, GF; Weiss, RG; Berger, RD; Lima, JA; Halperin, HR. Magnetic resonance assessment of the substrate for inducible ventricular tachycardia in nonischemic cardiomyopathy. *Circulation*, Vol. 112, (2005), pp 2821–2825, ISSN 1524-4539

Pacifico, A; Hohnloser, SH; Williams, JH et al. Prevention of implantable defibrillator shocks by treatment with sotalol. d,l-Sotalol Implantable Cardioverter-Defibrillator Study Group. *N Engl J Med*, Vol. 340, (1999), pp 1855–1862, ISSN 1533-4406

Pratt, CM; Al-Khalidi, HR; Brum, JM et al. Cumulative experience of azimilide associated torsades de pointes ventricular tachycardia in the 19 clinical studies comprising the azimilide database. *JACC*, Vol. 48, (2006), pp 471–477, ISSN 1558-3597

Raitt MH. Implantable Cardioverter-Defibrillator Shocks: A double-Edged Sword? *JACC*, Vol. 51, (2008), 1366-1368, ISSN 1558-3597

Raymond, JM; Sacher, F; Winslow, R; Tedrow, U; Stevenson, WG. Catheter ablation for scar related ventricular tachycardias. *Curr Probl Cardiol*, Vol. 34, (2009), pp 225-70, ISSN 0146-2806

Reddy, VY; Neuzil, P; Taborsky, M; Ruskin, JN. Short-term results of substrate mapping and radiofrequency ablation of ischemic ventricular tachycardia using a saline-irrigated catheter. *JACC*, Vol. 41, (2003), pp 2228–2236, ISSN 1558-3597

Reddy, VY; Reynolds, MR; Neuzil, P et al. Prophylactic catheter ablation for the prevention of defi brillator therapy. *N Engl J Med*, Vol. 357, (2007), pp 2657–65, ISSN 1533-4406

Reiffel, JA. Drug and drug-device therapy in heart failure patients in the post-COMET and SCD-HeFT era. *J Cardiovasc Pharmacol Ther*. Vol. 10, (Suppl 1), (2005), pp S45–S58, ISSN 1940-4034

Rosenqvist, M; Beyer, T; Block, M; Minten, J; Lindemans, F. Adverse events with transvenous implantable cardioverter-defibrillators: a prospective multicenter study: European 7219 Jewel ICD Investigators. *Circulation*, Vol. 98(1998), pp 663–670, ISSN 1524-4539

Santangeli, P; Di Biase, L; Dello Russo, A; Casella, M; Bartoletti, S; Santarelli, P; Pelargonio, G; Natale, A. Meta-Analysis: Age and Effectiveness of Prophylactic Implantable Cardioverter-Defibrillator. *Ann Intern Med* , Vol. 153, (2010), pp 592-599, ISSN 1539-3704

Soejima, K; Stevenson, WG; Sapp, JL; Selwyn, AP; Couper, G; Epstein, LM. Endocardial and epicardial radiofrequency ablation of ventricular tachycardia associated with dilated cardiomyopathy: the importance of low-voltage scars. *JACC*, Vol. 43, (2004), pp1834–1842, ISSN 1558-3597

Steinbeck, G; Dorwarth, U; Mattke, S et al. Hemodynamic deterioration during ICD implant: predictors of high-risk patient. *Am Heart J*, Vol. 127, (1994), pp 1064–1067, ISSN 1097-6744

Stevenson, WG; Khan, H; Sager, P; Saxon, LA; Middlekauff, HR; Natterson, PD; Wiener, I. Identification of reentry circuit sites during catheter mapping and radiofrequency ablation of ventricular tachycardia late after myocardial infarction. *Circulation*, Vol. 88, (1993), pp1647–167, ISSN 1524-4539

Stevenson, WG; Friedman, PL; Kocovic, D; Sager, PT; Saxon, LA; Pavri, B. Radiofrequency catheter ablation of ventricular tachycardia after myocardial infarction. *Circulation*, Vol. 98, (1998), pp 308 –314, ISSN 1524-4539

Stevenson, WG; Wilber, DJ; Natale, A; Jackman, WM; Marchlinski, FE; Talbert, T; Gonzalez, MD; Worley, SJ; Daoud, EG; Hwang, C; Schuger, C; Bump, TE; Jazayeri, M; Tomassoni, GF; Kopelman, HA; Soejima, K; Nakagawa, H. Multicenter Thermocool VT Ablation Trial Investigators. Irrigated radiofrequency catheter ablation guided by electroanatomic mapping for recurrent ventricular tachycardia after myocardial infarction: the multicenter thermocool ventricular tachycardia ablation trial. *Circulation*, Vol. 118, (2008), pp 2773–2782 ISSN 1524-4539

Stevenson WG. Preventing centricular tachycardia with catheter ablation. *Lancet*, Vol. 375, (2010), pp 4-6, ISSN 1470-2045

Tanner, H; Hindricks, G; Volkmer, M; Furniss, S; Ku¨hlkamp, V; Lacroix, D; de Chillou, C; Almendral, J; Caponi, D; Kuck, KH; Kottkamp, H. Catheter ablation of recurrent scar-related ventricular tachycardia using electroanatomical mapping and irrigated ablation technology: results of the prospective multicenter Euro-VT-study. *J Cardiovasc Electrophysiol.*, Vol 21, (2010), pp 47-53, ISSN 1532-2092

Tedeschi, CG & White, CW Jr. A morphologic study of canine hearts subjected to fibrillation, electrical defibrillation and manual compression. *Circulation*, Vol. 9, (1954), pp 916–21, ISSN 1524-4539

Torp-Pedersen, C; Moller, M; Bloch-Thomsen, PE et al. Dofetilide in patients with congestive heart failure and left ventricular dysfunction. Danish Investigations of Arrhythmia and Mortality on Dofetilide Study Group. *N Engl J Med*, Vol. 341, (1999), pp 857-865, ISSN 1533-4406

Trouton TG, Allen JD, Adgey AAJ. Oxidative metabolism and myocardial blood flow changes after transthoracic DC countershock in dogs. *Eur Heart J*, Vol. 13, (1992), pp 1431–40, ISSN 1522-9645

Van Vleet, JF; Tacker, WA Jr; Geddes, LA; Ferrans, VJ. Acute cardiac damage in dogs given multiple transthoracic shocks with a trapezoidal wave-form defibrillator. *Am J Vet Res*, Vol. 38(1977), pp 617–26, ISSN 0002-9645

Verma, A; Kilicaslan, F; Schweikert, RA; Tomassoni, G; Rossillo, A; Marrouche, NF; Ozduran, V; Wazni, OM; Elayi, SC; Saenz, LC; Minor, S; Cummings, JE; Burkhardt, JD; Hao, S; Beheiry, S; Tchou, PJ; Natale A. Short- and long-term success of substrate-based mapping and ablation of ventricular tachycardia in arrhythmogenic right ventricular dysplasia. *Circulation*, Vol. 111, (2005), pp 3209 - 3216, ISSN 1524-4539

Volkmer, M; Ouyang, F; Deger, F; Ernst, S; Goya, M; Ba¨nsch, D; Berodt, K; Kuck, KH; Antz, M. Substrate mapping vs. tachycardia mapping using CARTO in patients with coronary artery disease and ventricular tachycardia: impact on outcome of catheter ablation. *Europace*, (2006), pp 48–976, ISSN 1099-5129

Vorperian, VR; Havighurst, TC; Miller, S et al. Adverse effects of low dose amiodarone: a meta-analysis. *JACC*, Vol. 30, (1997), pp 791–798, ISSN 1558-3597

Waldo, AL; Camm, AJ; deRuyter, H et al. Effect of d-sotalol on mortality in patients with left ventricular dysfunction after recent and remote myocardial infarction. The SWORD Investigators. Survival with oral d-sotalol. *Lancet*, Vol. 348, (1996), pp 7–12, ISSN 1470-2045

Wathen, MS; DeGroot, PJ; Sweeney, MO et al., for the PainFREE Rx II Investigators. Prospective randomized multicenter trial of empirical antitachycardia pacing versus shocks for spontaneous rapid ventricular tachycardia in patients with implantable cardioverter-defibrillators. Pacing Fast Ventricular Tachycardia Reduces Shock Therapies (PainFREE Rx II) trial results. *Circulation*, Vol. 110, (2004), pp 2591-2596, ISSN 1524-4539

Wilber, DJ; Kopp, DE; Glascock, DN; Kinder, CA; Kall, JG. Catheter ablation of the mitral isthmus for ventricular tachycardia associated with inferior infarction. *Circulation*. Vol. 92, (1995), pp 3481–3489, ISSN 1524-4539

Wilson, CM; Allen, JD; Bridges, JB; Adgey, AAJ. Death and damage caused by multiple direct current shocks: studies in an animal model. *Eur Heart J* Vol. 9, (1988), pp 1257–65, ISSN 1522-9645

Worck, R; Haarbo, J; Thomsen, PEB. Electrophysiological study and 'slow' ventricular tachycardia predict appropriate therapy: results from a single-centre implantable cardiac defibrillator follow-up. *Europace*, Vol. 9, (2007), pp 1048-1053, ISSN 1099-5129

Zhan, C; Baine, WB; Sedrakyan, A; Steiner, C. Cardiac device implantation in the United States from 1997 through 2004: a population-based analysis. *J Gen Intern Med.*, Vol. 23(Suppl 1). (2008), pp 13–19, ISSN 0884-8734

Zhou L, Chen BP, Kluger J, Fan C, Chow MSS. Effects of amiodarone and its active metabolite desethylamiodarone on the ventricular defibrillation threshold. *JACC*, Vol. 31, (1998), pp 1672–1678, ISSN 1558-3597

Zipes, DP; Camm, AJ; Borggrefe, M; Buxton et al. (2006). ACC/AHA/ESC 2006 guidelines for management of patients with ventricular arrhythmias and the prevention of sudden cardiac death: a report of the American college of cardiology/American heart association task force and the European society of cardiology committee for practice guidelines (Writing committee to develop guidelines for management of patients with ventricular arrhythmias and the prevention of sudden cardiac death): developed in collaboration with the European heart rhythm association and the heart rhythm society. *Circulation*, Vol. 114(10), pp e385–e484, ISSN 1524-4539

7

Just in Time Support to Aide Cardio-Pulmonary Resuscitation

Frank A. Drews and Paul M. Picciano
University of Utah / Aptima Corp.
United States of America

1. Introduction

Cardiovascular disease is the leading cause of death in the United States with over 696,000 cases recorded by the Center for Disease Control (CDC) in 2002 (National Center for Health Statistics, 2002). In particular, Sudden Cardiac Arrest (SCA) claims 300,000 to 400,000 American lives annually (AHA, 2005, Huikuri, Castellanos & Myerburd, 2001, Zipes & Wellens, 1998). Ventricular fibrillation is believed to be the insidious perpetrator associated with the majority of these heart maladies (AHA, 2005, Cummins & Hazinski, 2000). Unfortunately, most victims that experience SCA have only a small chance of survival (Stiell, Nichol, Wells, De Maio, Nesbitt, Blackburn, & Spaite, 2003; Zipes & Wellens, 1998).

Increasing the probability of survival of SCA victims requires skilled and knowledgeable responders. Usually the task falls to EMTs, firefighters, police officers, or other highly trained responders. Unfortunately, these experts are not always available on site which means that critical time is lost by moving responders to the victim. An alternative approach to provide rapid access to responders is to develop and provide supportive technology that guides a novice through the procedure of resuscitating the victim by presenting information and feedback at the time when it is needed. However, such approach needs methodologically and conceptually to be rooted in cognitive psychology and human factors since these fields can direct work that aims at the robust improvement of human performance of novices. The successful application of this approach has the potential to improve usability of medical devices for non-experts, beyond the design of defibrillators.

Below we will outline the elements that need to be included in the development of a system that allows an untrained responder to deal with a SCA by providing elementary cardiopulmonary resuscitation (CPR). This approach is based on the idea of Just-in-Time Support (JITS). First, we will outline the tradition into which such JITS falls conceptually. Then, we will describe the differences between current architectures of Intelligent Tutorial Systems (ITS) and the constraints under which a true JITS has to operate. In the following section we provide a conceptual framework that allows analysis of human performance in the context of complex procedural tasks. Next, we will describe a JITS developed for the purpose of evaluating the feasibility and effectiveness of this approach, and report the results of an experimental study that evaluated a JITS. Finally, we will discuss the findings in the context of future developments of defibrillators and other systems that require guidance of novice users when using these advanced medical technologies in emergency situations.

1.1 Intelligent Tutorial Systems (ITS)

1.1.1 Description of ITS

Intelligent Tutoring Systems (ITS) have been developed over the last decades. Early systems focused on supporting students in acquiring knowledge, thus these systems were similar to flash cards but were also capable of analyzing a student's responses (Uhr, 1969). The next generation systems were more sophisticated because they moved from a scripted hierarchical structure of knowledge towards systems that were able to deal with potentially all requests that a student would submit to the system. For example SCHOLAR (Carbonell, 1970) tutored students in South American geography and was designed to deal with a variety of questions that might be asked by a student learner. The next important step in the development of ITS was embodied in the work of Collins (1977). Earlier that decade Craik & Lockhart (1972) demonstrated that deeper, more elaborate processing improved learning and retention. In application of this line of reasoning, Collins (1977) implemented a Socratic method of exploration for his system. What was remarkable about this approach was that it allowed the student to "discover" knowledge, empowering the student to acquire knowledge from experience and individual cases, through self-directed exploration of the knowledge base. Despite the wide range of ITS there are a number of basic elements that all of these systems have in common. These elements will be outlined next.

Many ITS projects share a basic architecture consisting of the same components. Perhaps the most basic components as described by Burns and Capps (1988) are the "Expert Model", the "Student Model" and the "Tutor". These modules are essential to the development of the JITS framework and will be discussed in depth.

Expert Model. The expert model is designed to encapsulate all available knowledge for a particular domain. Domains for which ITS's have been developed included arithmetic – BUGGY (Brown & Burton, 1978), programming language - LISPIT (Anderson, 1988), and electronic troubleshooting – SOPHIE (Brown, Burton, and deKleer, 1982). Clearly, it is a challenge to develop an expert model for an ITS and the difficulty is a function of how well defined a domain is. For example, when dealing with technical procedures like maintaining an aircraft, the problem space is well understood, i.e., the steps involved in performing a procedure are clearly structured and the means to perform the task are well defined. Clearly less well understood domains provide a significantly higher challenge for the designer of the expert model, and with Anderson (1988) one has to emphasize that, ". . . a great deal of effort needs to be expended to discover and codify the domain knowledge" (p.22). The information contained in the expert model is usually assembled by experts in specific fields and serves as the standard to which the student's actions and knowledge is compared.

Student Model. The student (or user) model is the system's representation of a specific learner's abilities and knowledge concerning the domain under consideration. Because of the dynamic nature of learning, a single or a static student model is not sufficient in an ITS. This is because overall the student acquires knowledge during the use of the system and progesses towards the development of expertise, but this track is not linear and perturbations of the user's proficiency across and even within a training session need to be accommodated. A critical function of ITS is to properly diagnose the user and identify when and what type of assistance is needed. If students perform below their normal baselines, the system must respond according. For the system to accurately gauge a student, it must go beyond a simple comparison to the expert model. One issue of current diagnostic functions implemented in ITS's is that they evaluate response accuracy by comparison with the knowledge base (Linn, 1990; Marshall, 1990). This allows for the categorization of a student, but offers nothing to guide learning and performance (Linn, 1990). However, the tutor model serves this purpose.

Tutor Model. The tutor model is essential in a ITS since it incorporates the didactic ideas of the designer. Without a tutoring model (e.g., instructional module, or pedagogical agent) an ITS would be limited to the administration and scoring of tests lacking the ability to impart knowledge or understanding to the user. Structurally, the instructional module interacts with the expert model and the student model to formulate relevant information to the user. It evaluates the student model in terms of the expert model and decides what information to present, how to display the information, and when to do so. The tutor model is the visible module for the user. Through the interface, the pedagogical agent serves as the teacher, consultant, assistant, or coach.

1.1.2 Limitations of ITS

The above description of the ITS architecture illustrates some of strength of the approach that guides the development of an ITS. However, there are also limitations that are associated with the development and use of such system. These limitations become particularly salient when the goal is to design a system that does not provide knowledge, but that can be used as a just-in-time support system. Certainly, both systems have similarities– e.g., both are primarily aimed at novices, are computer based, and leverage best practices of expert systems and user-interface principles. However, for the current purpose it is also critical to understand the differences between these systems. The differences can be described with regard to the goals, the time available for performance, the intended cognitive processing strategies and the system input. A brief summary of these issues is provided in Table 1, and will be discussed in detail in the next sections.

Objectives. The disparate objectives of each system are yoked to the temporal constraints associated with their use. With the ITS, the extended time horizon enables the goals of learning, long-term retention and fosters accuracy in the speed-accuracy trade-off. This situation can be contrasted with the JITS that is not focused on learning, since retention is inconsequential and potentially counter-productive in situations where a JITS is being used. The objective is to allow the user to perform the task to a satisfactory degree in the limited time available. Due to the temporal constraints, it is more important to sufficiently complete all requisite steps in the given, limited time rather than to strive for flawless performance on some tasks while failing to complete others.

Paradigm	Objectives	Time Available	Processing Strategies	System Input
Intelligent Tutoring Systems	Long term retention Learning Accuracy over speed	Long time horizon Self paced Low time pressure	Deep/elaborative Adaptive, transferable Declarative	Passive collection Requires user input to computer
Just-in-Time Support	Short term performance Complete task Speed over accuracy	Short time horizon Externally paced Significant time pressure	Shallow /perceptual Mimicking Procedural	Active collection Monitors user actions

Table 1. Differences between Just-in-Time Support (JITS) and Intelligent Tutoring Systems (ITS) on critical dimensions.

Time available. A student using an ITS to acquire some knowledge will not experience time pressure. The user determines the start time, duration, and sets the pace of the interaction with the system. This more relaxed situation can be contrasted with the context in which a JITS is being used. Here, the task will be subject to considerable time pressure due to the task criticality (a non-critical task could tolerate awaiting the arrival of an expert), making the task externally, and not internally paced. The JITS user operates under a limited time envelope in which to perform the task.

Processing strategies. A significant discrepancy between systems is also evident in the targeted cognitive processes involved in performance. The aim of an ITS is to target a deeper level of processing (Craik & Lockhart, 1972) which allows long term retention. Thus, intelligent tutoring systems utilize declarative knowledge permitting extensive mental associations and abstractions. This more elaborative processing strategy serves not only long-term retention, but also pliant, adaptive application with the development of domain expertise. In contrast a JITS targets a shallower, perceptual level of information processing. As a consequence, mimicking-type strategies, though inferior to elaborative processing for memory, are efficient for accomplishing procedural tasks without any previous practice in the task.

System input. The final difference concerns the input mechanisms that are implemented in each system. Traditional ITS requires a direct manipulation by the user (i.e., type, point and click, etc.). The system itself is designed to be passive whereas a JITS is specifically designed to actively collect data from the environment in which the task is performed. Equipped with an array of sensors the JITS system identifies changes of state and updates its models based on those changes. This process is implemented in such way that it is transparent to the operator (sensors are integrated with the tools used), and overall drives updated cues and feedback that guide performance to meet standards that suffice. Feedback and plan adaptability consequentially rely upon the external data the system is able to collect and integrate. The operator is permitted to act in a goal directed manner on the world (essential for performing a task), and is not required to provide additional information necessary to update the system's representation of the environment and the task progress.

Clearly, there are significant differences between the traditional ITS approach and the JITS design. One of the additional differences relates to the challenge of assessing performance of a human operator. To do this, a control theoretical perspective as proposed in the COCOM model can be useful. In the next sections we will describe this framework.

1.2 COCOM as conceptual framework

Erik Hollnagel (1993) developed the Contextual Control Model (COCOM) that describes a continuum of human control and can serve JITS development in both design and evaluation of operator performance. The model provides designers with a tool to identify parameters and determine control characteristics of an operator, which not only enables prediction of control conditions, but also establishes means to manipulate control states. Additionally, the model provides an effective assessment tool to evaluate performance hypotheses.

Before the nominal control modes can be described it is important to explain the parameters that characterize a given state of control of an operator. Based on Holnagel's model it is possible to distinguish several dimensions that help characterize the level at which a person is performing a control task. *Determination of outcome* is a reflection of an operator's ability to detect and interpret a change in system state. The *subjectively available time* is a measure that assesses the time pressure that is subjectively perceived by an operator. The *number of simultaneous goals* reflects the number of objectives the user can maintain concurrently and their relevance to the overall goal. The *availability of plans* is an expression of the controller's access to heuristics, plans, procedures or something rule-like to guide actions that are performed to accomplish the overall goal. The *event horizon* is composed of the extent to which previous information on the control task is being utilized in a given decision, plus the "prediction length", which is an extrapolation of the future state of the system. Finally, the *mode of execution* is a reflection of the overall way how an operator performs the control task. Two modes are possible, a "subsumed" (ballistic or feed forward) mode where actions are executed automatically. This mode requires assumptions and predictions with regard to the dynamics of the controlled system. The second mode is a "feedback" mode in which data of the tasks' state and progress guide future actions because a constant assessment of performance changes the guidance that is provided.

1.2.1 Control modes

The control continuum that describes the level of control of an operator is anchored by an absence of control at one end of the continuum, and highlights several milestones as control progresses to a very high-level of control at the other end of the continuum. Hollnagel identified four characteristic regions of control. From the level of least control to level of greatest control the regions are labeled: *scrambled, opportunistic, tactical,* and *strategic* levels of control. A more detailed description of these levels with regard to the dimensions outlined above will be provided next.

The level of *scrambled* control resides on the lowest end of the continuum, and is an expression of a lack of control of the operator. The user performs the next action at random and the choice of action is unpredictable, resulting in a trial and error approach with limited determination of the outcome. Here, this approach results in user actions being incongruous with the situation. Clearly, a user operating in a scrambled control mode has no knowledge about the process and lacks any heuristics, rules or procedures that would allow performing the task. Consequentially, the user experiences a great deal of stress due to high cognitive workload, time pressure, and a futile understanding of the system and/or the current environmental conditions.

The *opportunistic* level of control is the next region on the continuum of control. What is important at this level is the fact that the operator expresses some ability to move the system toward the overall goal state. Similar to the scrambled mode of control, the operator still perceives significant time pressure, but it is possible for the user to plan the next action that is being performed. In addition, actions are no longer characterized by chance. Overall these changes are a reflection of the fact that control now becomes a cognitive problem, i.e., control is based on the user's ability to recognize and act on salient cues in the environment and that are provided by the system. Thus, the operator moved from a subsumed mode of execution to a feedback based mode, with feedback being accessible and interpretable and the environment being somewhat familiar.

A the level of *tactical* control a noticeable change in perceived time pressure occurs which allows for short range planning. The user experiences an expansion of the event horizon that is involved in planning, in both directions (previous states and predicted states). Performance now is based on previously acquired rules or procedures and the operator is now in a position where it is possible to anticipate needs associated with the control task that are in the near future. The meanings of the outcomes of actions are more completely understood, and two or three goals the operator pursues may be active at once, with a plan, rule, or procedure supporting each of the goals. Feedback is an important input and being utilized for comparison with higher level goals.

Finally, the *strategic* level of control is a state of high stability and planning that is well beyond the immediate context of the control task. Performance at this level is effective and robust with the event horizon being further extended in both directions. The operator has the opportunity to contemplate the highest level goals and performs at both modes of execution (i.e., feedback and feed forward control). Finally, performing at the strategic level of performance requires substantial motivation to do so. The user must embrace the high cognitive load associated with this level of performance that is a result of extended planning, reasoning, and observation to attain a strategic mode of control. Because of this high cognitive demand, strategic control often cannot be maintained for long periods. A summary of the different modes of control and their association with the different COCOM parameters is displayed in Table 2.

Parameters	Scrambled	Opportunistic	Tactical	Strategic
Determination of Outcomes	Obscured	Limited	Context dependent	Elaborate + prediction
Subjective Time Pressure	Severe	Significant – Severe	Light-Moderate	None
Simultaneous Goals	0-1	1	2-3	2-many
Availability of Plans	None employed	Minimal	Most goals supported by plans	Plans and contingencies available for all
Event horizon	Present only	Some history, little planning	Planning (based on current situation), use of previous data	Extensive planning & use of historic data
Mode of Execution	Subsumed	Feedback	Feedback	Feedback + subsumed
Action Selection	Random	Cue driven	Plan driven	Prediction driven

Table 2. Summary of COCOM parameters and control states (adapted from Hollnagel, 1993).

One important aspect with regard to the different modes of control is related to how an operator can switch between these modes. Below we will discuss the process of transitioning between modes.

1.2.2 Mode transitions

The transition between control modes is also of importance, and can be discussed in terms of changes in the parameters outlined above. Since those characteristics describe a state of control, it is appropriate to speak about an operator moving along the control continuum as result of a change in one or more of those parameters.

The most direct transition is a simple step to an adjacent level of control. This shift may be either an increase or a reduction of control performance. However, it is possible to have transitions that skip a level. For example, an operator in a tactical control mode may encounter a completely novel crisis. During such encounter the subjectively available time may diminish and no heuristics for employment are available. Clearly, a scrambled condition has resulted. Hollnagel (1993) insists that there is a constraint in moving to and from strategic control with strategic control only being reached from the tactical region and also only be able to degrade to the tactical level.

Knowing the characteristics of each control mode, allows identifying the region in which an operator is performing. Knowledge of the task, tools, and context permits a developer of a system to articulate mode control predictions which provide a workspace that can be manipulated in an effort to improve an operator's level of control. For example, one implementation is to make accessible a plan to a user where the person did not have any previously. In addition, it is possible to rectify the absence of salient features by providing guidance. Finally, clear feedback can be presented to promote interpretation that can guide action.

Lastly, the application of COCOM as a model of human performance provides some guidance for the development of assessment tools of human performance in the context of complex tasks, i.e., the assessment of performance using a JITS system. Thus, Hollnagel's model provides valuable characteristics to describe the task and desired performance which can allow prediction of performance in a given situation.

1.2.3 Design considerations based on COCOM

After the above description and analysis of the COCOM model it is now possible to identify several important design recommendations. These recommendations guided the implementation of the Just-in-Time System to provide CPR expertise. Below each of these principles is outlined.

- Provide a plan of action to the user that is adaptable to dynamic conditions and needs
- Provide salient, action-directing cues to the user
- Provide easily interpretable feedback to help the user correct actions and update system state continuously
- Work within time constraints that are derived from the task.

Clearly any direction provided to a user of a JITS needs to include the visual and auditory modality to provide instructions and feedback. Visual displays can inform a novice on how to proceed when performing individual steps of the task. This implies that a dynamic visual display has to

- demonstrate sequential actions in a procedural task
- obtain attention focused on specific tasks or presentation displays
- illustrate a task which is difficult to describe verbally
- represent invisible system functions or behaviors in a transparent fashion.

1.3 Additional design considerations

1.3.1 Expertise

A substantial amount of research has been conducted to identify what characterizes expert behavior and expert performance (e.g., Chi, Glaser, & Farr, 1988,). Glaser and Chi (1988) established seven general attributes representative of experts. These attributes are presented in table 3.

1.	Experts excel in their own domain.
2.	Experts perceive large meaningful patterns.
3.	Experts solve problems quickly with little error.
4.	Experts have superior short- and long-term memory in their domains.
5.	Experts represent problems more abstractly.
6.	Experts are able to spend great deal of time analyzing a problem qualitatively.
7.	Experts have strong self-monitoring skills.

Table 3. Expert characteristics (Glaser & Chi, 1988).

1.3.2 Expert-novice differences

Johnson (1988) observed that novices do not have extensive domain knowledge, and cannot encode information well (e.g. they lack an adequate representation and experience pattern matching difficulties) nor process new information quickly. Miller & Perlis (1997) also discussed novices' inferior knowledge base and structure, adherence to superficial cues, and utilization of small, fragmented information units. Not only did novices utilize more superficial knowledge, but the knowledge base lacked cross referencing and the organization that experts are able to impose.

In developing a system for non-experts it is of critical importance to understand the limitations of novices. This can lead to an implementation of guidance that truly supports performance but does not exceed novices' abilities. Below are the design recommendations pertinent to each expert characteristic described in Table 3.

- Novices do not excel in the given domain, they need help. Thus, there is a need for JITS.
- Novices need to parse information into simpler, more digestible chunks. Critical parameters and combinations must be salient. The system helps the user to construct patterns in small increments.
- The pace at which information is delivered to novices should be slowed. Information about sequential steps may also need altering. Repetitions in displaying this information may be necessary. The pedagogical model should monitor and control the pace and sequence pursuant to operator needs.
- The system should relieve burdens to short term and long term memory of novices by holding the information and making it visible, accessible, and congruent with the current subtask.
- Novices do not understand abstract concepts of the domain. Cues and feedback must utilize concrete representations. Designers cannot assume knowledge on the part of the user. Metaphors, higher level concepts, and domain knowledge are likely to be lost on a novice.
- Novices will not have time or ability to analyze the situation on a deeper level. A context-aware system will be responsible for identifying the proper course of action.
- Novices will likely be far too stressed to have any resources available to deal with the challenges required in building situation comprehension. Smart algorithms and sensors take over this job in conjunction with the situation assessment the system monitors operator performance in order to optimize cues and feedback to assist the user optimally.

The emphasis in employing these design recommendation is that it is imperative to provide information congruent with the operator's knowledge. For the development of an effective system it is important to design systems that are suited for the user's level of expertise. It also is important to not attempt to transform novices into experts when developing JITS systems since acquisition of expertise exceeds available time. Often, tasks may consist of a single trial, which is clearly not sufficient to establish expertise. However, by abandoning the effort to create an expert and embracing the task of mimicking one, several advantages arise. For example, a shallow level of information processing can be targeted. Certainly such level of processing is inferior for retention, but it reduces the demand on the novice's limited cognitive resources and leverages more primitive processes such as perception-action mechanisms. To summarize the following design principles with regard to expertise need to guide the development of a JITS:

- Break information down into comprehensible chunks
- Use concrete (as opposed to abstract) representations
- Ensure the pace of information delivery is apt for user population
- Minimize cognitive burdens (memory, search, attention capture) as much as possible.
- System should assume monitoring role
- Keep information visible

1.3.3 Feedback

Feedback can be defined as information that is provided to an operator that is relevant in the context of assessing performance or outcomes. In order to provide closed-loop control, feedback must be communicated directly to a user, and if provided correctly it has the potential to enhance operator control.

Numerous reviews and meta-analyses demonstrated the effectiveness of accurate feedback in a variety of tasks (Azevedo & Bernard, 1995, Kluger & DeNisi, 1996, Salmoni, Schmidt, & Walker,1984). Reliable feedback enhances learning and performance. In support of immediate task facilitation, Goodman (1998) concluded that frequent and immediate feedback to study participants improved performance during practice. Similarly, Young & Lee (2001) found that more feedback in the "acquisition phase" facilitated task performance (but not retention). In JITS supported tasks, "practice" occurs simultaneously with the "test". Therefore, frequent and immediate feedback will likely generate desired effects for JITS systems. An additional benefit of feedback is that it increases motivation. Participants often invest more effort, show more interest in the task, and persist longer than those who do not receive feedback. Interestingly, Salmoni, Schmidt, & Walker (1984) found these effects persisted for some time even after removing feedback.

Based on the above, a number of recommendations for optimal delivery of feedback in a JITS can be provided:

- Customize feedback pursuant to operator knowledge
- Feedback provided must be reliable
    1. Conflicting information can confuse the user
    2. Excess precision (based on user knowledge) will likely be ignored
- Feedback timing is critical
    1. User must be able to relate feedback to relevant activity
    2. User must be ready to attend to feedback information
- Feedback may serve as motivation in completing the task

1.3.4 Visual displays

Since most of the tasks supported by JITS entail spatial arrangements, information needs to be presented visually to the user. Technology-intense domains typically require visual displays to support detection and interpretation of events, particularly when governed by capricious constraints (Sanderson, Haskell & Flach, 1992). This assessment certainly applies to the CPR/defibrillation task. Park and Hopkins (1992) outlined six conditions in which dynamic visual displays (DVDs) are effective. The majority of those conditions are highly cogent with JITS system development to support CPR. The use of DVDs is effective when:

- Demonstrating sequential actions in a procedural task
- Obtaining attention focused on specific tasks or presentation displays
- Illustrating a task which is difficult to describe verbally
- Explicitly representing invisible system functions or behaviors.

Based on the above the following design recommendations for dynamic visual displays can be used in the context of JITS development:

- Important for conveying dynamic visuo-spatial information which is often difficult to verbalize
- Appropriate for sequencing and procedural information
- Effectively portray motion and trajectory
- Animations should be simple and relevant
- Pacing of dynamic visuals must be carefully considered

1.4 JITS framework

After the previous sections outlined the design recommendations for a JITS, in the next sections the JITS framework will be presented.

1.4.1 Real time support

Because the primary application of a JITS system is in the context of performing urgent tasks without the user of the system having task expertise available, system based support needs to be provided in real-time. With the task being one of urgency, any implementation has to address the fact that performance is under high time pressure and the time horizon of the task is short.

The main purpose of the JITS system is to support performance of a user by structuring the instructions in such way that they can be easily followed, even by a complete novice. This goal is accomplished by breaking down the overall task into its elements or sub-tasks and by presenting these sub-tasks individually to reduce the cognitive load that is imposed on the user of the system (see section 1.3 for design recommendations).

Because the JITS systems' focus is on short term performance and immediate task completion, it supports the user with the goal to mimic an expert without the necessity of long-term retention which is the main focus of intelligent tutorial systems. This goal is achieved by adaptive information presentation. This information presentation approach aims at supporting shallow, perceptual processing of the information that enables the user to mimic the displayed procedures to a level of proficiency that meets minimal performance standards. The goal can be achieved through effective information presentation (see section 1.3 for design recommendations).

1.4.2 Information presentation

Visualization of information is optimal for conveying complex, temporally constrained, spatial information. In many cases, a task will require a space-dependent manipulation of the environment through effectors such as tools or direct contact. According to Schmidt and

Kaysor (1987) who report the superiority of simple graphics compared to photographs, a simple graphical presentation can lead to superior information processing (see also Harrison, 1995). Further, displaying information based largely on graphics and animation can transcend language-induced barriers. Though, if language is not likely to be a concern, the combination of graphics and text produces superior results to either alone (Booher, 1975).

Animation has the advantage of allowing the novice to mimic expert behavior simply through observation. For example, Palmiter and Elkerton (1991) found that participants using animation performed training session tasks in approximately half the time required of a text using group and this without sacrificing accuracy! In training, the animation group surpassed the text group by performing over 90% of their trials correctly, while the text-based group failed to achieve 80% correct. The findings suggest that participants in the animation group adopted a mimicking strategy.

A JITS system's real-time support displays manual/technical aspects of the subtasks by showing animations of how and where to perform a task (e.g., tilting the head of the victim) and instructs how to attach the sensors. After attaching sensors to a patient, the system provides real-time feedback about the patient's vital signs and offers context dependent suggestions for the next step of the treatment protocol. This reduces the cognitive load and eliminates the requirement of planning next steps that are conditional on current situation assessment.

1.4.3 Adaptive support

Another important implication of the task setting under which a JITS can be maximally effective is that the speed at which the task needs to be performed and the sequence of the sub-tasks is determined externally. This implies that changes in the environment need to have a direct impact on the selection and execution of procedures by the user. The basic idea of a JITS is that it addresses these requirements by providing adaptive support to the user. Adaptive support is possible because the system collects continuously data in the task environment by using advanced sensor technology. The collected data are then used to provide context specific instructions that can lead to performance that addresses the problem at hand optimally. Support for this approach is provided by Carlson, Lundy, and Schneider (1992) who report evidence that guidance is effective in supporting novices when dealing with novel tasks where long-term retention is not required. Guidance also supports a novice by taking advantage of the hierarchically structured task that is the basis for any task that can be implemented using a JITS. This structure allows the presentation of information in the exact order that is needed to execute the procedure optimally (see Bovair & Kieras, 1991; Jansen & Steehouder, 1996).

The JITS system guides the user by providing a plan that effectively provides the novice operator with the expertise necessary to successfully perform the task. However, as JITS will have to accommodate novices, it is important to understand the differences and communalities of information requirements for experts and novices. There are important differences in information requirements between experts and novices that are based on the different cognitive representations used by the two groups during task performance. For example, experts tend to think more abstractly, perceive meaningful patterns, and organize tasks based on their domain expertise (Chi, Farr, & Glaser, 1988). In contrast, novices are less likely to reason and organize abstractly in the domain, fail to recognize patterns, and rely on concrete representations (Miller & Perlis, 1997). Thus, simply transmitting expert knowledge to novices is likely to yield errors.

Overall, in the context of the current JITS system user guidance is implemented as context dependent recommendations about the next step in the procedure that needs to be taken to achieve satisfactory performance. In addition, the system supports decision making at decision points in the protocol by highlighting the correct protocol branch. Novice decision-makers tend to be overwhelmed when provided with multiple alternatives. By highlighting the recommended course of action the cognitive load is reduced and no alternatives have to be evaluated requiring careful assessment of the current situation.

A schematic overview of the Just-In-Time system that was evaluated in the experimental study is illustrate in Figure 1 below.

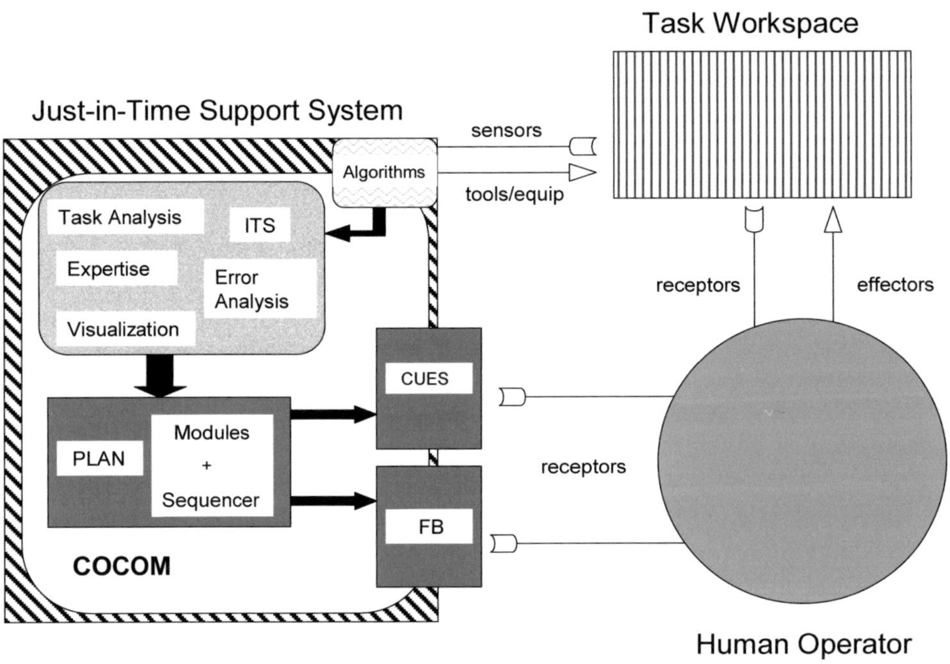

Fig. 1. Schematic of a Just-in-Time Support System.

2. Methods

The experimental study used a randomized 3 (training) x 2 (device) nested factorial design. Naïve participants received one of three training programs and returned 2 weeks later to complete the experimental procedure in one of the two conditions (either with or without device assistance). Device-based sensors collected multiple measures providing means to analyze participant performance during the assessment phase.

2.1 Participants

A total of 100 participants took part in the study. The participants were largely members of the University of Utah community. The mean age for participants was 22.6 (SD=6.7) years. Because of the focus of the study, it was a requirement that participants did not have knowledge in CPR or first aid. Forty-five participants claimed prior CPR training with a mean of 6.5 years (SD=6.5) since the training (it is common that high school students from the area receive a training class however, it does not result in certification). A questionnaire was administered with the goal to screen for the extent of CPR knowledge. The researchers asked if participants had been trained in CPR or with an AED and asked basic skill questions such as the ABCs of CPR. None of the participants was able to answer all of the knowledge questions correctly. Correct answer of all of the simple questions would have resulted in exclusion from participation in the study.

2.2 Training

Three different training conditions were utilized in the experiment. The "CPR" training consisted of a slightly modified version of the American Heart Association (AHA) protocol. The modifications included dropping portions of the procedure including checking for pulse and calling for help as these were not emphasized in the present study. Two groups of twenty (total 40) participants received CPR training. Twenty (20) more participants received "device" training (*DEV-DEV* in Table 4) mirroring CPR training and incorporating the device into the instruction process. A registered nurse administered the CPR and device training. Prior to completing the training, each individual demonstrated aptitude to an adequate level and trained to criteria. Finally, two more groups (20 per group) trained in a fashion unrelated to the task. The experimental design called for two control groups in which no task relevant training was given. These participants learned strategies to improve verbal scores on the graduate record examination (GRE). *Table 4* provides a visual representation of the design and names the groups according to experimental condition.

N=100		**no device**	**device**
Training	**CPR trained (n=60 total)**	*GRE-NO (n=20)*	*CPR-DEV (n=20) / DEV-DEV (n=20)*
	GRE trained (n=40 total)	*GRE-NO (n=20)*	*GRE-DEV (n=20)*

Table 4. Experimental Design.

2.3 Apparatus

The JITS device aims at providing a means for novice users to perform effective CPR and defibrillation tasks. Based on the American Heart Association (AHA) protocol from 2006, the device delivered instructions crafted for novice understanding via visual and auditory prompts. Utilizing smart sensors and algorithms, the device assessed user actions and customized feedback to guide and ultimately improve performance. For example, if the sensors detected the chest compressions were too shallow and too slow, it prompted the user to "push harder" and "push faster" for the next set of compressions. The sensors not only drove feedback algorithms but also collected data on task performance. In addition to relieving many cognitive burdens, there were also engineered improvements such as the integrated headrest and mask. Pre-experiment investigation revealed many novice responders had difficulty maintaining an open airway while giving breaths. The headrest was designed to ensure victim head-tilt to keep the airway open without requiring the responder to manually perform the task each time while giving breaths. *Figure 2* shows the device in use.

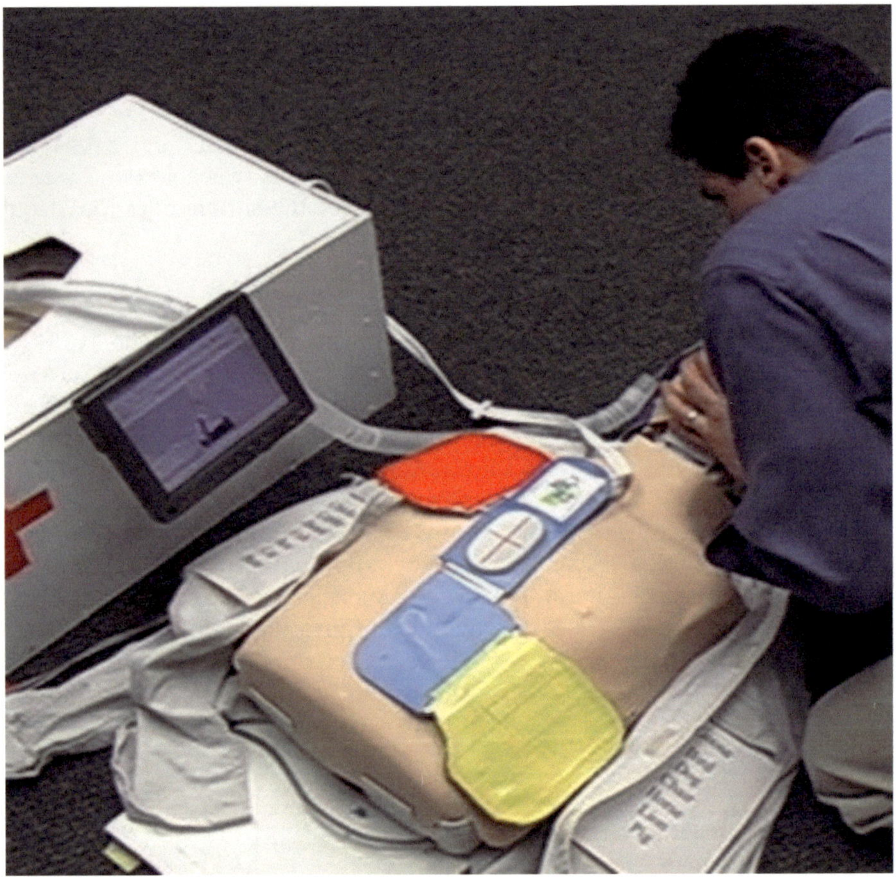

Fig. 2. The device in use on training mannequin.

The system provided the first visual and auditory cues to initiate the actions of the novice responder. The system governed the pace and content in accord with the operator performance by monitoring changes in the task space (i.e. tool placement, flow meter readings). For example, the instructions required for rescue breaths were withheld until the system recognized correct head placement. Pressure sensor in the headrest determined the placement of the victim's head. The system managed the action plan and provided the user simple, actionable commands.

After giving simple instructions and monitoring performance, the system then provided feedback if necessary. For example, after placing the mask, the system stated 'give two breaths" and provided an animation demonstrating the proper method. Then the sensors actively monitored the inspired volume of air into the lungs. If the rescuer delivered insufficient volumes, instead of moving to the next step, the system encouraged the responder to "give two large breaths". Feedback of this kind was critical in elevating and stabilizing performance early in the scenario.

A headrest, anesthesia breathing mask (with one-way valve), and defibrillator pads from Zoll's AED-plus®, and Lilliput® 8-inch touch screen LCD served as the tools available to the responders in the "device" condition (Figure 3.). The headrest was customized from foam. Two pressure sensors were inserted at the neck and in the center of the bowl of the headrest (in order to detect proper head placement). The mask apparatus consisted of a standard anesthesia mask, bacteria filter and a one-way valve (directs victim's exhalation away from the responder).

A desktop and a laptop computer provided the computing resources for generating the displayed animations and auditory cues as well as collecting data from: two Novametrix Medical Systems, Inc. CO_2SMO Plus flow monitors (one inside the mannequin, a second externally in the mask); pressure sensors (headrest), and linear potentiometer placed on the spring inside the mannequin.

The signals collected from the sensors were converted by a PMD 1208 LS, Measurement Computing Systems analog-to-digital converter. All software was written in C++. A Laerdal Medical Little Annie® mannequin portrayed the victim for each responder. The mouthpiece was exchanged and discarded for every responder while the bacteria filter and mannequin "lungs" were replaced every five participants or fewer as needed.

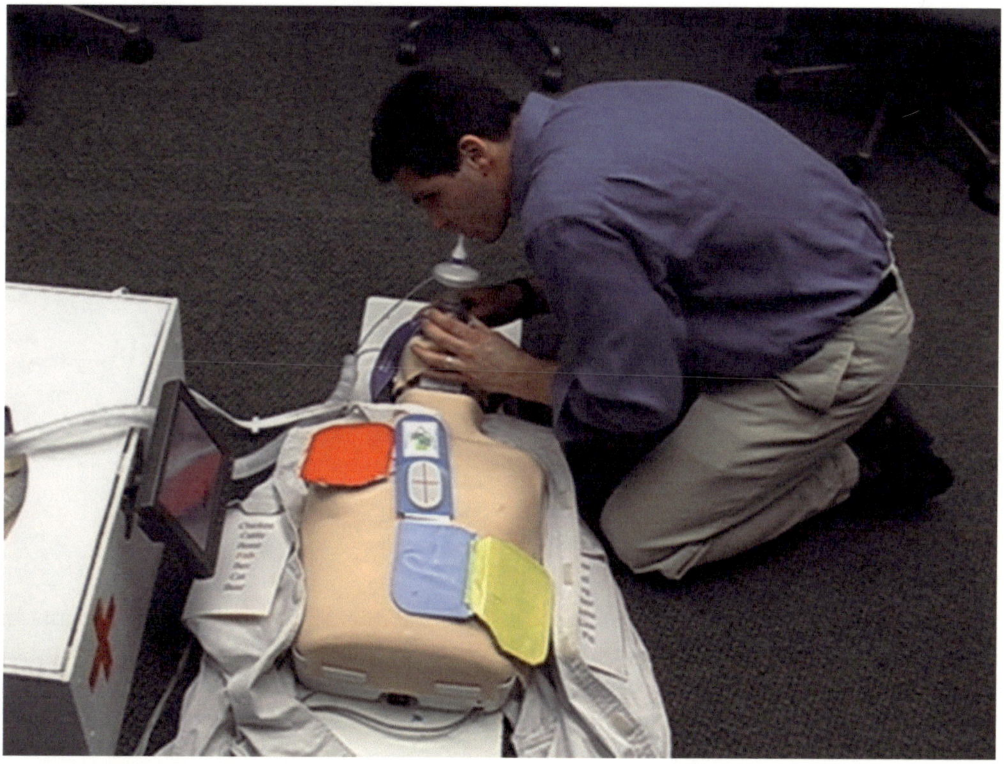

Fig. 3. Components of the device.

2.4 Procedure

Training sessions were offered at various times and locations for a period of 90 days. Participants were blinded to the type of training they would undergo. After the group training session, each individual was to schedule a testing date a minimum of fourteen days to a maximum of twenty-one days after training. Participants' self selection of training and experimental times contributed to the randomization process.

Upon returning for the experimental session the experimenter ensured consent forms were completed, verified previous training, and read the participant the appropriate instructions. All participants were informed that they would enter a room with an unconscious victim (no breathing, no pulse). Their task was to perform CPR until help arrived (the victim would remain unconsciousness for the entire scenario).

The groups that were not utilizing the device were informed that "tools" would be available adjacent to the victim. These included a mask for ventilating the victim as well as pads associated with the defibrillator. The components were identical to those available in the device condition.

The device group had the added benefit of the headrest and of course, the protocol, audio and visual cues and feedback presented by the device. Pre-experiment instructions encouraged device-group participants "...to follow the instructions of the device as closely as possible". A still frame of the video instruction to place the headrest is displayed in *Figure 4*.

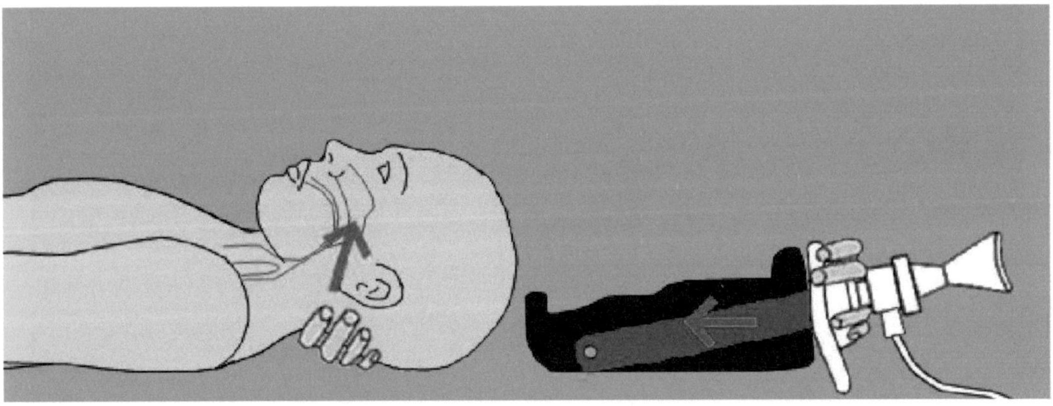

Fig. 4. Screenshot of video instruction "place headrest".

After completing the scenario, the researcher praised the efforts of the participants and reassured them it was simply a simulation with an inanimate object. The debriefing also included a survey to assess actions and a number of variables that based on COCOM should be sensitive to differences between groups. Finally participants were thanked for their time and paid $30.

2.5 Coder training

Research assistants coded participant behavior based on a number of categories for each of the steps of performing the task of providing CPR. Participant activities were coded as falling into one of the categories based on Hollnagel's COCOM model.

	Control mode (COCOM)		
	Scrambled	**Opportunistic**	**Tactical**
Mask	no two hand use of mask	Two hand use, with effective seal	Two hand use (anesthesia based) with effective seal
Breaths	audible leak	give when system commands	look for chest rise while giving
Chest compressions	One handed; wrong grip	Chest compressions with beeps	15 consistent chest compressions (despite beeps)
Body	excessive move (waist shoulders)	looks @ screen	little movement to accomplish
Verbal comments by participants	"what"/"how to do ....?"; expression of frustration	Comments expressing insights e.g., "Oh", "Ahh"	count out loud; articulate plan
Start/Stop	begin action- without finish (correct)	system interrupt; follow system	ignore system to perform correct
Tools	fail to use; explore; search; can't find immediately	used on command	use correct without prompt anticipate
Pads	don't use pads at all	watch screen for placement of pads	place pads without looking at screen; correct placement before or without cue or feedback

Table 5. Coding of performance based on COCOM.

2.6 Post experimental questionnaire

To identify group based differences on subjective measures like action selection, utilization of cues and feedback, determination of outcomes, goal setting, and time pressure a post-experimental questionnaire was applied. For example, to assess the perception of feedback in the scenario participants were asked to rate on a 10 point scale how effective feedback was ranging from a value of 1 – I did not receive feedback to a value of 10 – feedback was helpful. The basic assumption is that participants in the different experimental conditions should be sensitive to differences in manipulation based on predictions from COCOM and these differences should be reflected in measures like action selection, utilization of feedback, determination of outcomes, goal setting and subjective time-pressure since they are sensitive to the level of control of a participant.

3. Results

3.1 Control modes

Four trained coders who were blinded to the hypotheses of the study performed the control mode analyses. After each coder succeeded in a 4 hour training that familiarized them with the categories and their definitions, they were tested on example videos that represented samples of the observation study. Each coder was trained until they reached 95% accuracy of detecting and coding behavior as specified in the definitions. Next, in a different session they were instructed on how to review the video recordings and who to record their observations to the data sheet. Inter-rater reliability was assessed with Cohen's Kappa (Kappa = 0.899). This kappa value is well above the commonly accepted 0.70 level threshold validating the use of the coding results.

Table 2 summarizes the proportion of actions by mode for each participant group. A multivariate analysis of the control mode data resulted in a significant difference for experimental group (Wilks'Lambda = 0.049, approximate F(12, 246.3) = 43.6, p < 0.001). Next univariate and post-hoc Scheffe tests were conducted to analyze the overall finding in more detail. The results of these analyses are discussed in the sections below.

Group	%Scrambled	%Opportunistic	%Tactical
GRE-NO	90(12)	4(7)	5(7)
GRE-DEV	30(15)	66(15)	4(8)
CPR-NO	19(22)	16(7)	64(25)
CPR-DEV	17(12)	62(16)	21(17)
DEV-DEV	15(9)	60(10)	24(12)

Table 6. Group means for COCOM classification (in percent). Standard deviations in parentheses.

In a comprehensive analysis that categorized participants as being in a particular mode of control based on the median of their actions falling within one of the three control modes, all of the participants in the *GRE-NO* group were classified as performing in the scrambled control mode at the aggregated level. A more detailed analysis of the average percentage of actions across the group and not based on individuals falling into one of the three control modes revealed that almost all of the actions of participants in this condition were classified as displaying scrambled behavior (M = 90%, SD = 12%). Post-hoc comparisons revealed the 90% mean for *GRE-NO* was significantly higher compared to scrambled mode scores for all other groups (p < 0.001) (see Figure 5).

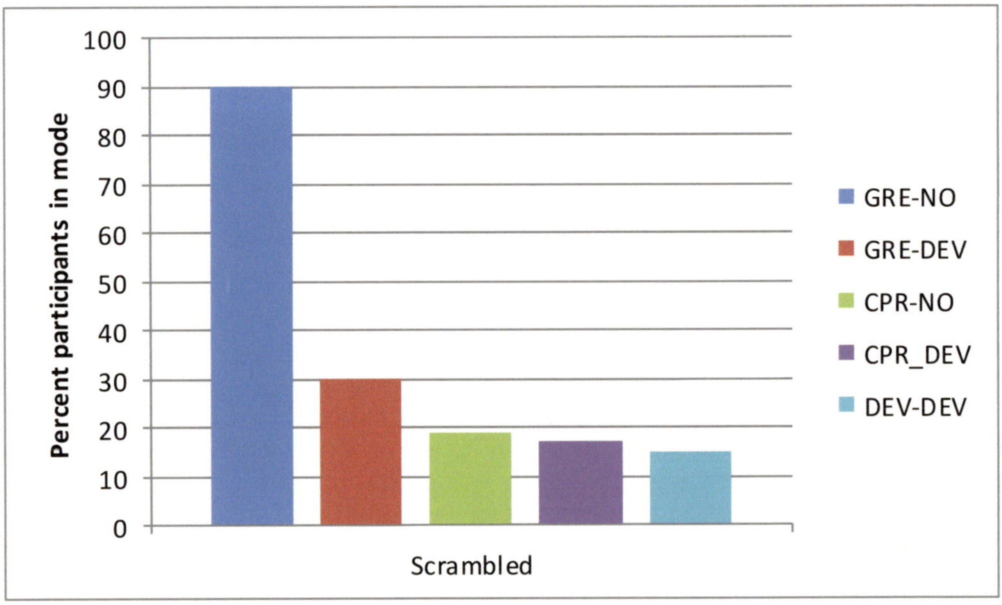

Fig. 5. Scrambled control mode for all experimental conditions.

In contrast to the *GRE-NO* group of participants, participants in the *GRE-DEV* condition benefited from the provisions of plans, cues, and feedback and demonstrated an opportunistic control mode. Overall, only two participants (10%) in this group were classified as acting at the scrambled level of behavior, while all other participants in this group performed in an opportunistic mode of control. In a more detailed analysis focusing on individual actions, the *GRE-DEV* group posted the highest proportion of opportunistic behaviors (M = 66%, SD =15%) (see *Figure 6*). Post-hoc tests demonstrated that this percentage was significantly higher than the two non-device groups ($p < 0.001$) but not statistically different from the other two device groups ($p \geq 0.658$). Most of *GRE-DEV*'s remaining actions (M = 30%, SD = 15%) resembled a scrambled mode of control (see *Figure 5*).

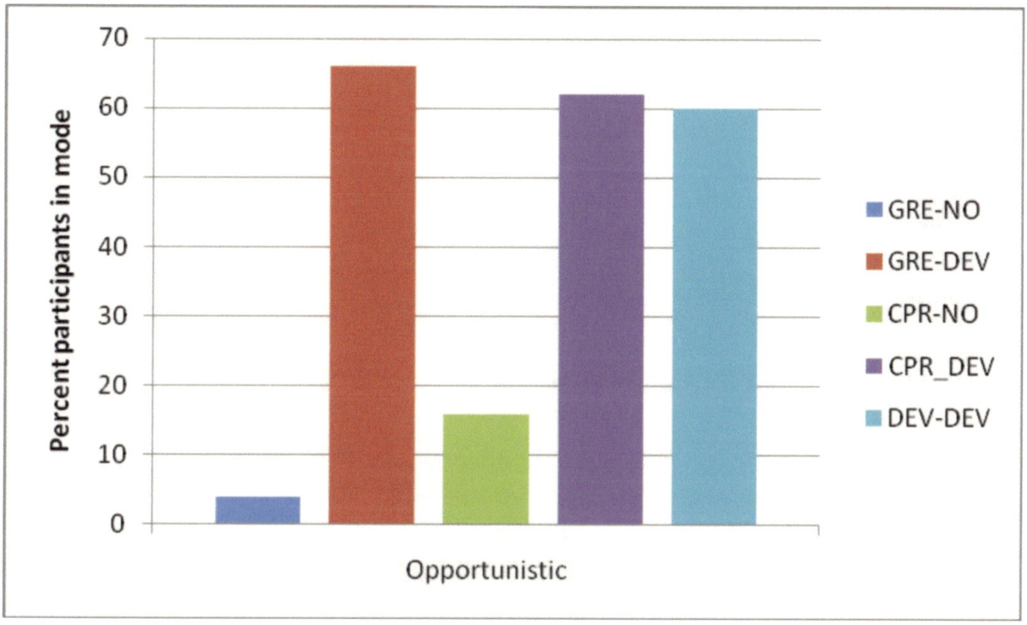

Fig. 6. Opportunistic control mode for all experimental conditions.

The *CPR-NO* group consisted of well trained but unsupported (no plan, cues, or feedback) participants, relying on knowledge retrieval based on their previous training to perform the task. Adequate performance given the background of participants should facilitate a tactical control mode, which is supported by the data (*Figure 7*). Overall of the twenty participants in the *CPR-NO* group, eighteen were classified as acting at the tactical level, and only two participants were coded as performing at the scrambled level of control. When analyzing individual actions at the group level, actions that were classified as being representative for tactical control accounted for the majority (M = 64%, SD = 25%) of their activity, which is significantly higher than any other group ($p < 0.001$). In addition, this group's opportunistic control mode score (M = 16%, SD = 7%) was significantly lower than the three device groups ($p < 0.001$), and the *CPR-NO's* scrambled score (M = 19%, SD = 22%) was comparable to the three device groups and reveals that participants in all groups made some errors when performing the task.

The device clearly captured participant's attention in the *CPR-DEV* group where 16 participants' actions were classified as falling into the opportunistic mode of control, three participants were classified as acting in the tactical control mode, and one participant was performing in the scrambled control mode. Again, the three device groups did not differ significantly in their opportunistic scores ($p \geq 0.658$), nor scrambled scores ($p \geq 0.074$), but *GRE-DEV* did lag the other two groups in tactical actions ($p \leq 0.026$).

Finally, analyzing the performance in the *DEV-DEV* group revealed that at the aggregated level, all 20 participants in *DEV-DEV* group were classified as performing at the opportunistic mode of control. This overall performance is also reflected in the fact that the analysis of individual actions revealed that the majority of actions were performed at the opportunistic control mode, approximately 20 % of the actions were performed in the tactical control mode, and the fewest number of all actions of all groups was performed in the scrambled mode of control.

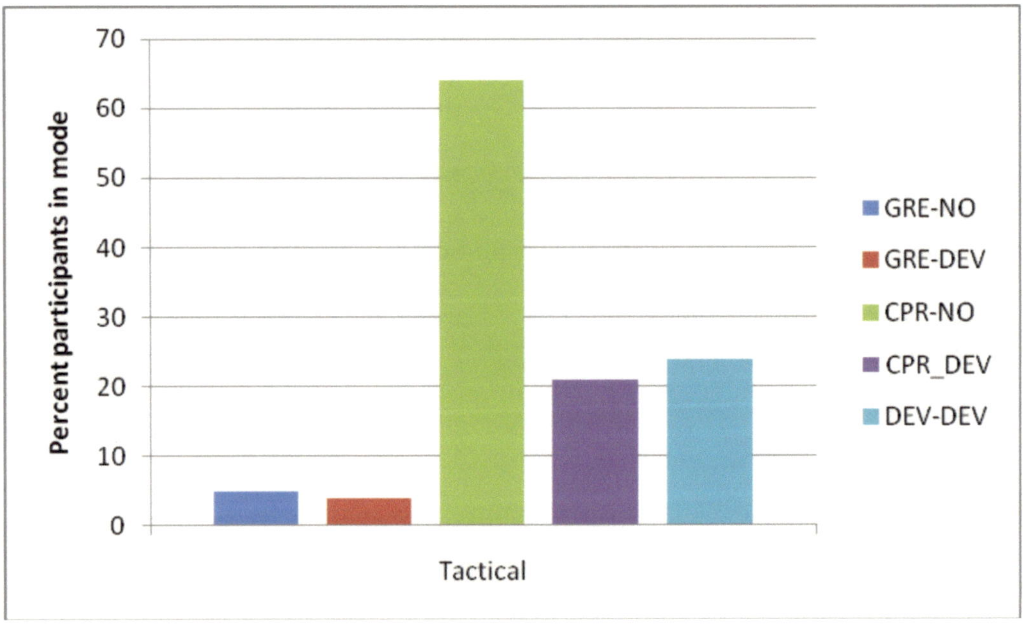

Fig. 7. Tactical control mode for all experimental conditions.

3.2 Protocol compliance

Another analysis focused specifically at the subtasks that were classified as necessary to comply with the American Heart Association's CPR protocol. Specific comparisons between each experimental condition were performed to identify the degree of compliance with these steps. For this purpose, the number of correctly completed steps achieved by each participant was recorded. The analysis was confined to only the first cycle of providing CPR since one of the constraints of these tasks is that all tasks must be completed the first time through the procedure. For example, if the pads are placed in the first cycle, there is no need to complete that step in each cycle. Subsequently, only a subset of the tasks was repeated.

Again, two trained coders (same training procedure as described above applied) independently evaluated each action on the video recordings and determined if participants correctly completed the required nine activities. Of the 900 judgments, only 19 discrepancies between the coders emerged resulting in high concurrence between the raters (agreement exceeded 97.8%). *Table 7* contains the number of protocol steps each group performed correctly.

Experimental group	**GRE-NO (GRE training - no device)**	**GRE-DEV (GRE training - device)**	**CPR-NO (CPR training - no device)**	**CPR-DEV (CPR training - device)**	**DEV-DEV (device training - device)**
MEAN	1.6 (1.46)	7.80 (1.05)	7.85 (1.49)	8.45 (0.88)	8.65 (0.49)

Table 7. Mean number of protocol steps executed correctly (9 max) standard deviation in parentheses.

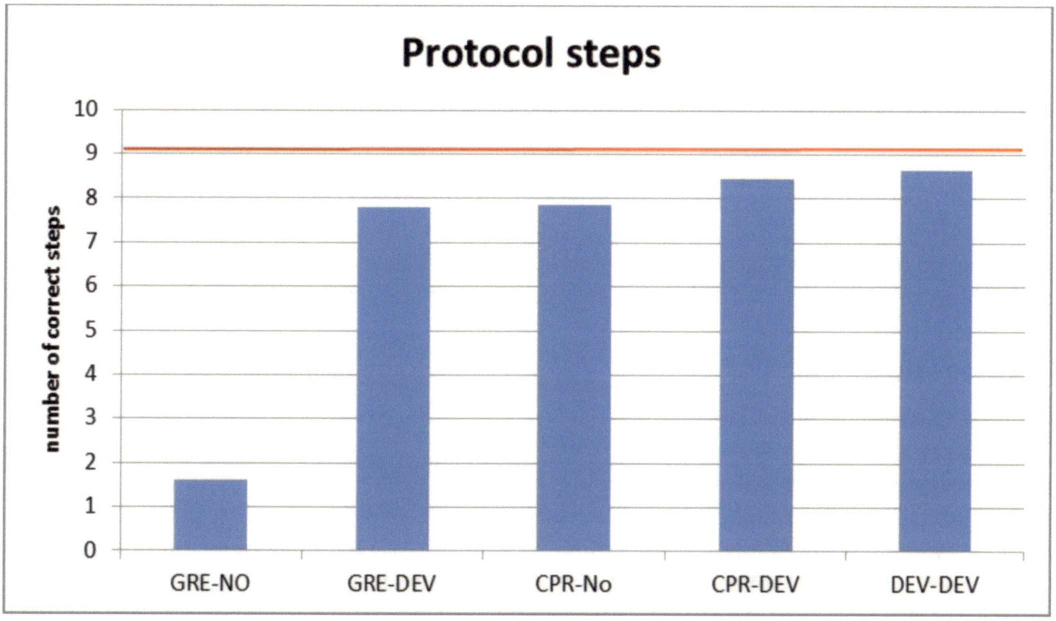

Fig. 8. Average number of correctly performed steps in accordance with the AHA protocol for each experimental condition. The red line indicates perfect performance.

Statistical analyses revealed that the group means were significantly different ($F(4,95) = 135$, $p<0.001$) overall (see Figure 8). Post-hoc comparisons indicated that the *GRE-NO* was unable to accomplish most subtasks that are critical to CPR and defibrillation ($p < 0.001$). Interestingly, there was no difference in performance between any of the other four experimental groups. All of these groups were able to complete the required steps at a level of performance that is statistically not different. Finally, inspection of the standard deviation for each group indicates that the DEV-DEV had the smallest level of variation, where GRE-NO and CPR-NO had high levels of performance related variability between participants within each group. Overall, this descriptive finding indicates that external guidance in the DEV-DEV supported standardization of performance, where the two groups that had no such guidance available were more heterogeneous in terms of compliance with the AHA required steps.

3.3 Post experimental survey data

The post-experimental questionnaire served as yet another instrument employed to assess the bounds of control mode categories and provided converging evidence for the hypothesis that the different experimental conditions lead to differences in control mode. The survey instrument utilized multiple scales to represent different COCOM parameters. Specifically, scales represented action selection, utilization of cues and feedback, determination of outcomes, for goal setting, and time pressure. The inquiries concerning action drivers (includes cues), feedback utilization, and outcome determination yielded results consistent with hypotheses

In general, participants in the *GRE-NO* condition exhibited a scrambled control mode as they reported no use of *feedback* and minimal determination of the *outcome*. Participants in the *GRE-DEV* condition showed a high reliance on *cues* and *feedback* where participants in the *CPR-NO* condition ranked *feedback* very low and recorded the highest *action* score avowing their use of a memorized plan to drive their actions. All of these findings are consistent with predictions based on COCOM. However, inconsistent with COCOM predictions the survey results concerning subjective time pressure were not supportive of COCOM predictions. According to the COCOM, operators in scrambled mode have a proclivity to perceive an enormous limit of the time for action available, however, there was no difference between groups ($F<1$). The lack of a difference between groups can potentially be attributed to the fact that the scenario length was relatively high (more than 5 minutes). Thus the available time may have subjectively felt as being sufficient and superseded any time pressure participants may have experienced at the start of the scenario.

4. Discussion

4.1 COCOM and JITS

The vision of the JITS framework is to provide guidance for the development of systems that are capable of enhancing user performance as operators confront unfamiliar tasks that require immediate intervention by a task novice. Based on the findings of the present study there is support for the idea that the JITS accomplishes this challenge by providing adaptive plans, cues, and feedback tailored to the user's understanding. System flexibility is required to adapt to dynamic contextual conditions as well as user behavior.

The basis for the COCOM-derived dependent measures reside in Hollnagel's mode characteristics. Each of the subtasks when providing CPR (i.e. holding mask, placing pads, delivering compressions) provided subtleties for control mode classification. For example, one technique for holding the mask was the anesthesia-style hold taught in training. This grip exemplified tactical control as it demonstrated knowledge retention and skill.

Overall, the *GRE-NO group* performed 90% of their actions in scrambled mode. All 20 participants coded as scrambled overall for the scenario. Based on the fact that they had neither skills nor knowledge to employ, there was little probability they could perform in any other manner. The *CPR-NO* group demonstrated tactical control a majority of the time (64%). However, their erroneous behavior was highlighted by 20% of their actions being coded as scrambled and 60% of the responders failing to properly sequence the subtasks. Examining the device groups, *GRE-DEV* was hypothesized to demonstrate opportunistic control and the data of this study support that claim. Sixty-six percent of the actions of participants in this group were coded as opportunistic. Participants also made some mistakes as evidenced by 30% of their actions classified as scrambled. Observation of their performance indicated that many of the mistakes occurred early in the scenario. Anecdotal examples include some confusion while searching for the mask, and giving compressions with the wrong grip and compressing much more slowly than the required pace. Most device-aided participants corrected their actions in the subsequent CPR cycles after receiving feedback.

Trained groups using the device also demonstrated control profiles easily adapted to the COCOM paradigm. At first glance, their training should have enabled them to demonstrate some tactical mode characteristics. Nonetheless, the presence of the system would likely drive their actions in the direction of opportunistic control. The question to be determined empirically was related to the proportion of opportunistic to tactical methods. Each *trained-device* group performed roughly 20% - 25% of their actions in tactical mode and more than 60% in opportunistic. Two factors are most plausible for generating this distribution. First, the system was explicitly designed to seize attention and engage the operator throughout the scenario. Second, with what can be considered limited training and practice, most operators would likely defer to the system for expertise.

In general, *GRE-NO* exhibited a scrambled control mode as they reported no use of *feedback* and minimal determination of the *outcome*. *GRE-DEV* showed a high reliance on *cues* and *feedback*. *CPR-NO* ranked *feedback* very low and recorded the highest *action* score avowing their use of a memorized plan to drive their actions. One disappointment in the survey results came from the *time pressure* scale. According to the COCOM, operators in scrambled mode have a proclivity to perceive an enormous limit of the time available. However, due to the length of the scenario and lack of purposeful activity, five minutes probably felt like a long time superseding any time pressure they may have experienced at the start of the scenario (it did to the researchers watching them struggle).

To conclude, there are many advantages to widespread deployment of such a system. The delay in getting professional responders to the scene is well documented. Precious moments are lost in transport. Additionally, it has been shown that even when they arrive, they are not performing optimally. Based on the results of the present study, it clearly is possible to develop novice supportive technology that is based on Human Factors principles. Such technology not only will be user friendly, for example support users to use defibrillators more effectively, but ultimately save lives.

The leading question of this work was, is it possible to identify indicators of performance that help understand how to better design systems that provide instructions at the time when need is greatest. Thus, after describing COCOM, we outlined the Just-in-Time Support framework, described an implementation of this framework in the context of providing CPR, and provided data in support of the hypothesis that human factors driven implementation of just in time support technology can guide performance of novices.

In addition, the present work represents one of the earliest applications of COCOM to generate dependent measures sufficiently robust for quantitative analysis. Very few researchers attempted to test COCOM predictions in such a manner largely due to the inchoate bounds of control modes and an inability to derive cogent measures. Stanton, Ashleigh, Roberts, and Xu, (2001) provided the first empirical support for COCOM hypotheses. However, the process of coding behavior was lacking some of the necessary rigor to allow generalizable inferences based on this work.

4.2 Conclusions

This work demonstrates in the context of a complex task that it is possible to develop Just-in-Time Systems that are capable of instructing a task novice in performing a task at a level that suffices in terms of outcomes. Clearly, this needs to be the main goal when the alternative is scrambled behaviour of a person without instruction or knowledge, that is likely to do more harm than good. In addition, there are a number of contexts where systems that follow the guidance of COCOM in determining how to effectively guide an operator can be of use. Among those context is certainly the use of defibrillators, and especially systems where guidance needs to be tailored to users who due to a number of factors (e.g., age) are not performing at the highest possible cognitive level and are in need of support.

5. References

American Heart Association. (2005). Heart Disease and Stroke Statistics — 2005 Update. Dallas, Tex.: American Heart Association; available at http://www.americanheart.org/presenter.jhtml?identifier=1928

Anderson, J.R., (1983). The architecture of cognition. Cambridge, MA: Harvard University Press.

Anderson, J.R. (1988). The expert module. In M. Polson & J. Richardson (Eds.), Foundations of Intelligent Tutoring Systems. Hillsdale, NJ: Lawrence Erlbaum Associates, Inc.

Azevedo, R. & Bernard, R.(1995). A meta-analysis of the effect of feedback in computer based instruction. Journal of Educational Computing Research, 13(2), 109-125.

Booher, H. (1975). Relative comprehensibility of pictorial information and printed words in proceduralized instructions. Human Factors, (17), 261-277.

Brown, J. S., Burton, R. R., (1978). Diagnostic models for procedural bugs in mathematical skills. Cognitive Science, 2, 155-191.

Brown, J. S., Burton, R. R., & deKleer, J. (1982). Pedagogical, natural language and knowledge engineering techniques in SOPHIE I, II and III. In D. Sleeman & J. S. Brown (Eds.), Intelligent Tutoring Systems. New York: Academic Press.

Burns, H.L., & Capps, C.G. (1988). Foundations in intelligent tutoring systems: An Introduction. In M. Polson & J. Richardson (Eds.), Foundations of Intelligent Tutoring Systems. Hillsdale, NJ: Lawrence Erlbaum Associates, Inc.

Carbonell, J.R. (1970). AI in CAI: An artificial intelligence approach to computer-assisted instruction. IEEE Transactions on Man-Machine Systems, 11(4), 190-202.

Chi, M.T.M., Glaser, R., & Farr, M.J (Eds.). (1988). The Nature of Expertise. Hillsdale, NJ: Erlbaum.

Collins, A. (1977). Processes in acquiring knowledge. In R. Anderson, R. Spiro, & W. Montague, (Eds.), Schooling and the acquisition of knowledge. Hillsdale, NJ: Lawrence Erlbaum Associates.

Craik, F. & Lockhart, R. (1972). Levels of processing: A framework for memory research. Journal of Verbal Learning & Verbal Behavior, 11, 671-684.

Cummins, R., & Hazinski, M.F. (Eds.)(2000). Guidelines 2000 for cardiopulmonary resuscitation and emergency cardiovascular care. Circulation. Vol. 102(8). Supplement I. August

Goodman, J. S. (1998). The interactive effects of task and external feeack on practice performance and learning. Organizational behavior and human decision processes, 76(3), December, pp.223-252.

Glaser, R. & Chi, M. T. M. (1988). Overview. In M. Chi, R. Glaser & M. Farr (Eds.), The Nature of Expertise (pp. xv-xxvii). Hillsdale, NJ: Erlbaum.

Graham, C., Scollon, D. (2002). Cardiopulmonary resuscitation training for undergraduate medical students: a five year study. Medical Education, 36, 296-298

Hollnagel, E. (1993). Human Reliability Analysis and Control. London: Academic Press

Huikuri, H.V., Castellanos, A., Myerburd, R. (2001). Sudden cardiac death due to cardiac arrhythmias. N Engl J Med, Vol. 345, No. 20

Johnson, E.J. (1988). Expertise and decision under uncertainty: Performance and process. In M. Chi, R. Glaser & M. Farr (Eds.), The Nature of Expertise. (pp. 209-228). Hillsdale, NJ: Erlbaum.

Kluger, A., & DeNisi, A. (1996). The effect of feedback interventions on performance: A historical review, a meta-analysis, and a preliminary feedback intervention theory. Psychological Bulleting, 119(2), 254-284.

Linn, R. L. (1990). Diagnostice testing. In N. Frederiksen, R. Glaser, A. Lesgold, M. Shafto (Eds.), Diagnostic Monitoring of Skill and Knowledge Acquisition (pp.489-498). Hillsdale, New Jersey: Lawrence Erlbaum Associates.

Marshall, S. P. (1990) Generating good items for diagnostic tests. In N, Frederiksen, R. Glaser, A. Lesgold, M. Shafto (Eds.), Diagnostic Monitoring of Skill and Knowledge Acquisition, pp.433-452. Hillsdale, New Jersey: Lawrence Erlbaum Associates, Inc.

Miller, M., & Perlis, D. (1997). Toward automated expert reasoning and expert-novice communication. In P. Feltovivh, K. Ford, & R. Hoffman (Eds.), Expertise in context (pp.405-415). Menlo Park, CA: American Association for Artificial Intelligence.

National Center for Health Statistics, data for 2002 (2005). National Vital Statistics Report Vol. 53. No. 17. available at http://www.cdc.gov/nchs/data/dvs/nvsr53_17tableE2002.pdf

Park, O., & Hopkins, R. (1992). Instructional conditions for using dynamic visual displays: A review. Instructional Science, 21(6), 427-449.

Sanderson, P., Haskell, I., & Flach, J. (1992). The complex role of perceptual organization in visual display design theory. Ergonomics, 35(10), 1199-1219.

Salmoni, A., Schmidt, R., & Walter, C. (1984). Knowledge of results and motor learning: A review and critical reappraisal. Psychological Bulletin, 95(3), 355-386.

Stanton, N., Ashleigh, M., Roberts, A., & Xu, F. (2001). Testin Hollnagel's contextual control model: Assessing team behavior in a human supervisory control task. International Journal of Cognitive Ergonomics, 5(2), 111-123.

Stiell, I., Nichol, G., Wells, G., De Maio, V., Nesbitt, L., Blackburn, J., & Spaite, D. (2003). Health-related quality of life is better for cardiac arrest survivors wh received citizen cardiopulmonary resuscitation. Circulation, 108, 1939-1944.

Uhr, L. (1969). Teaching machine programs that generate problems as a function of interaction with students. Proceedings of the 24th National Conference of Education, Virginia, April 2-4, 1969.

Young, D.E. & Lee, T.D. (2001). Skill Learning: Augmented feedback. In W. Karwowski (Ed.) International Encyclopedia of Ergonomics and Human Factors. (pp. 558-562). London: Taylor & Francis.

Zipes, D., Wellens, H.(1998). Sudden cardiac death. Circulation:98:2334-2351.

8

Electrical Storm in the Era of Implantable Cardioverter Defibrillators

David T. Huang[1] and Darren Traub[2]
[1]*Director of Cardiac Electrophysiology, University of Rochester Medical Center, Rochester, NY*
[2]*Cardiac Electrophysiologist, The Medical School at Temple - St. Luke's, Bethlehem, PA*
United States of America

1. Introduction

"Electrical storm" (ES) has been adopted as the term used to describe a period of cardiac electrical instability manifested by recurrent malignant ventricular arrhythmias. The definition of ES and the clinical implications of an episode have evolved as our armamentarium of pharmacologic, device -based and interventional anti-arrhythmic therapies has broadened. Prior to the widespread use of implantable cardioverter defibrillators (ICDs), the most commonly accepted definition of arrhythmia storm or electrical storm was "recurrent hemodynamically destabilizing ventricular tachycardia or ventricular fibrillation occurring two or more times in a 24-hour period, and usually requiring electrical cardioversion or defibrillation". [1-8] An episode of electrical storm carried serious clinical consequences with an in-hospital mortality rate of up to 14% during the first 48 hours.[3,6,7]. The mortality rate for an out-of hospital episode of electrical storm can only be speculated but would of course be similar to the 80-90% mortality rate of an out of hospital cardiac arrest[7-9].

Because ICDs often terminate potentially life threatening ventricular arrhythmias before any signs or symptoms of hemodynamic instability develop, the definition of ES has been modified and continues to be the subject of debate [12,8,-13]. Currently, the most widely accepted definition of ES in the literature and clinical practice is the occurrence of ≥ 3 distinct episodes of ventricular tachycardia (VT) and/or ventricular fibrillation (VF) within a 24-hour period resulting in device intervention (anti-tachycardia pacing [ATP] and/or shock delivery)[1,2,6,8,11-15]. To qualify as electrical storm, the three episodes of ventricular tachycardia or ventricular fibrillation cannot be continuous VT/VF in which device therapy is unsuccessful. Some authors have assigned an arbitrary time interval, generally 5-minutes between VT/VF episodes, as requisite in the definition of electrical storm[11-15]. Others have stated that incessant ventricular tachycardia or fibrillation, in which device therapy results in the return of even one beat of native rhythm should be included in the scope of ES, representing the most serious form of ES [1,2,8,11-15].

2. Incidence and timing of ES

The majority of data regarding the incidence, timing and prognosis of electrical storm comes from patients who have undergone ICD implantation for secondary prevention of cardiac arrest (table 1). Lack of a consensus definition for ES, as well as differences in ICD implant indications, concomitant medical therapy, and follow-up periods all contribute to the disparate reported incidence rates of 10-60% in the secondary prevention population. Using the definition of >/= 3 VF/VT episodes in 24-hours requiring device intervention, the incidence of ES is approximately 10-28% over a 1-3 year follow-up period when ICDs are placed for secondary prevention of cardiac arrest[1,2,8,10-21]. From a more consistent study population in the Multicenter Automatic Defibrillator Implantation Trial II (MADIT II), the reported incidence of electrical storm in a primary prevention ICD population is substantially lower at 4%[13].

Author	Definition	Incidence	Prognosis
Fries[22]	≥ 2 VT w/ 1 hr SR	60%, (34/57)	↑ in mortality over mean follow up 3y, 26% with ES vs 4% without ES (*P* < .05)
Credner[6]	≥ 3 VT/24 hr	10%, (14/136)	No ↑ in mortality
Greene[17]	≥ 3 VT/24 hr	18%, (40/227)	No ↑ in mortality
Bansch[15]	≥ 3 VT/24 hr	28%, (30/106)	RR 2.17 for mortality (CI 1.35 -3.48, *P* = .031)
Exner[12*]	≥ 3 VT/24 hr	20%, (90/457)	RR 2.4 for mortality (CI 1.3 -4.2, *P* = .03)
Verma[20]	≥ 2 VT/24 hr	10%, (208/2028)	↑ in mortality (*P* = .001, RR not listed)
Stuber[16]	≥ 3 VT/2 weeks	24%, (51/214)	5-y survival of 67% with ES vs 91% without ES (*P*=.0007)
Gatzoulis[14]	≥ 3 VT/24 hr	19%, (32/169)	RR 2.13 for mortality (CI 1.07 - 4.24, *P* = .031)
Hohnloser[18]	≥ 3 VT/ 24 hr	23%, (148/633)	No ↑ in mortality
Arya[19]	≥ 3 VT/ 24 hr	14%, (22/162)	N/A
Brigadeau[21]	≥ 2 Sep VT/24 hr	40%, (123/307)	No ↑ in mortality
Sesselberg[13†]	≥ 3 VT/ 24 hr	4%, (27/719)	RR 7.4 for mortality (CI 3.8 -14.4, *P*<.01)

*Secondary prevention population – AVID trial.
†Primary prevention population – MADIT II.
SR, sinus rhythm; VT, ventricular tachycardia; hr, hour; Sep, separate; RR, relative risk; CI, confidence interval

Table 1. Incidence and Prognosis of Electrical Storm.

The time from ICD implant to first episode of electrical storm varies among published reports. This heterogeneity of timing likely stems from differing device indications, cardiac substrate, and adjuvant medical therapy. In the series by Credner et al among patients whose ICDs were implanted for secondary prevention, 10% experienced electrical storm at a mean follow-up time of 4.4+/-4.5 months. This is the earliest reported time period from ICD implant to ES, but was similar to that of ICD implant to first appropriate device therapy of 4.1+/-4.8 months in this series[6]. Among 457 patients who received an ICD with advanced storage capability in the secondary prevention trial Antiarrhythmics Versus Implantable

Defibrillators (AVID), the incidence of storm was 20% with the initial episode occurring 9.2+/-11.5 months after ICD implantation[12]. A sub-study of the MADIT II trial, which represents the largest database to analyze ES in a primary prevention population, reported a 4% incidence of ES at a mean time of 11.1+/-9.4 months[13].

Frequent episodes of ventricular tachycardia can occur in the peri-operative period following ICD implantation. This was seen more commonly with open thoracotomy placement of epicardial patch electrodes than with newer transvenous ICD systems. The etiology of this peri-operative electrical instability is likely myocardial inflammation and treatment with standard anti-arrhythmic therapy is often ineffective[22-24]. An early increase in the incidence of ventricular arrhythmias has been reported in some patients with cardiac resynchronization devices. The mechanisms are as yet unclear but have been speculated to be related to increased dispersion of repolarization as well as gradients of concealment from differential ventricular pacing.[25-26]

3. Causes/triggers and risk factors for electrical storm

Among published reports an acute cause or trigger for electrical storm was identified in the minority of episodes. Even an exhaustive search for an acute cause may prove fruitless in up to 80% of patients.[1-3] The Shock Inhibition Evaluation with Azimilide (SHIELD) trial assessed the effects of azimilide on the frequency of device therapies in ICD patients. A precipitating cause for ES was found in only 13% (19/148) of storm patients in the SHIELD trial. The causes for ES were new or worsened congestive heart failure in 9% (13/148) and electrolyte disturbances in 4% (6/148)[18]. The usual suspect factors for precipitation of arrhythmias, such as electrolyte imbalance, ischemia, congestive heart failure (CHF) exacerbation and medication noncompliance, etc. have been reported with variable frequencies.[1,2,6,12-18] In a restropective review of 40 secondary prevention patients with a total of 61 electrical storms, Greene et al. reported no identifiable cause in 29%, new or worsened CHF in 15%, medication non-compliance or adjustment of antiarrhythmic medication in 20%, psychological stress in 10%, post-ICD placement in 13% and excess alcohol use in 8%.[18] The reported 70% identification of an acute cause in this series is disparate from the larger published trials but does point out the need to take a thorough history when presented with a storm patients to effectively treat the current storm episode and prevent further ES.

Of equal importance to recognizing acute precipitants of storm is identifying factors that would increase the risks for developing repetitive malignant arrhythmias in ICD patients. Secondary analysis of the MADIT II trial revealed that patients who had post-enrollment coronary events (myocardial infarction or angina) were 3.1 times more likely to experience electrical storm.[13] In fact, 7 (26%) of 27 patients with ES suffered an ischemic event within 4 weeks of their initial storm episode. Renal insufficiency was associated with a 2.1-fold increase in risk for electrical storm in the primary prevention MADIT II trial and has been associated with increased risk in secondary prevention populations[13,21] The clinical variable most strongly associated with development of ES among MADIT II patients was an interim post-enrollment arrhythmic event in the form of isolated ventricular tachycardia or ventricular fibrillation. Of the patients who experienced electrical storm during follow-up, 52% of them had a prior isolated arrhythmic event. These patients were 9.1 times more likely to experience electrical storm than patients without these isolated tachyarrhythmias.[13] Although interim hospitalization for congestive heart failure was predictive of appropriate device therapy for VT/VF in the MADIT II trial, it was not predictive of electrical storm.[13,27]

Data investigating acute causes of and risk factors for development of ES have often grouped together diverse patient populations with an array of cardiovascular substrates, degrees of CHF, revascularization status, ischemic burden, medical therapy and so on. Because of this, the literature to date is far from comprehensive or conclusive, but does imply that storm is the result of a complex interplay between a predisposing electrophysiological substrate and acute alterations in autonomic tone and cellular milieu. Dynamic progression of the underlying myocardial substrate through progressive tissue fibrosis, ischemia and/or ventricular remodeling can manifest as an isolated tachyarrhythmic episode heralding future electrical storm. The critical role of increased sympathetic activity in precipitating storm is substantiated by the temporal relation to worsening CHF, concurrent medical illness and emotional stress. [1,2,6,8,11-13,].

4. Arrhythmias and ICD therapies during electrical storm

The majority of storm episodes (86-97%) are caused by monomorphic ventricular tachycardia. VF alone accounts for 1%-21% of ES, mixed VT/VF 3%-14% and polymorphic VT 2-8%.[1,2,6,8-21] As illustrated in table 2, there is an extremely variable distribution in the number of tachycardias per episode of storm, as well as the number and types of therapies

StudyA	**ES Arrhythmias**	**No. of VT/VF episodes per ES**	**ES Therapies**
Fries[22]	Majority VT, percentages not listed	NA	43% with ATP only, 25% ATP and shock, 23% shock only
Credner[6]	64% VT, 21% VF, 14% VT+VF	Mean = 17 ± 17 (range, 3 to 50)	NA
Greene[17]	97% VT, 3% pVT	Mean = 55 ± 90 (range, 4 to 465)	23% with ATP only, 77% ICD shock ± ATP
Bansch[15]	86% VT, 8% pVT/VF, 4% VTs with various morph.	Median = 19 (range, to 440)	NA
Exner[12]	I86% VT, 14% VF or VT+VF	Median = 4 (range, 3 to 14)	46% shocks only, 28% ATP only, 26% shocks and ATP
Verma[20]	52% VT, 48% VF	NA	5 ± 5 shocks
Stuber[16]	93% VT, 7% pVT	Median = 8 (range, 3 to 1200)	31% ICD shock only, 19% ATP followed by shock, 50% ATP only
Gatzoulis[14]	NA	NA	ATP 21 ± 33 per ES episode Shocks 8 ± 4 per ES episode
Hohnloser[18]	91% VT, 8% VT+VF, 1% VF	Median =5 (range, 3 to 11)	7% ICD shock only, 70% ATP only, 23% shocks and ATP
Brigadeau[21]	90% VT, 8% VF, 2% pVT	Range = 2 to $\geq$ 15	18% shocks only, 26% ATP only, 56% shocks and ATP
Sesselberg[13]	78% VT, 22% VF	NA	NA

VT, ventricular tachycardia; pVT, polymorphic ventricular tachycardia; VF, ventricular fibrillation; ATP, anti-tachycardia pacing

Table 2. Arrhythmias and Therapies During Episodes of Electrical Storm.

delivered. The clinical presentation of storm can range from repetitive hemodynamically destabilizing episodes of VT/VF requiring multiple ICD shocks to asymptomatic tachycardias that are treated by ATP and discovered retrospectively through outpatient ICD interrogation. Whether patient outcomes are influenced by the clinical manifestations and therapies delivered during an episode of storm is unknown.[1,2,6,8-21]

Verma et al[20] , reported a significant correlation between the initial arrhythmia that led to ICD implantation and the arrhythmia responsible for ES. Among patients whose ICDs were placed for prior VT, 64% of ES episodes were caused by VT compared to only 28% by VF. For those patients whose ICDs were placed for prior VF, 45% of ES episodes were caused by VF and only 14% by VT.[20] Analysis of MADIT II patients with electrical storm revealed similar findings. Of 12 patients who had a prior episode of VT, 11 subsequently had VT as their initial rhythm in their ES. Patients with a prior isolated episode of VF also had this rhythm as their initial rhythm in the first ES.[13,20] The predilection for patients with coronary artery disease (CAD) and previous VT to have storm caused by monomophic VT, taken together with the influence of storm on future survival (discussed later), raises the question as to whether medical therapy alone is an aggressive enough strategy for prevention of ES in patients with ischemic cardiomyopathy who experience appropriate ICD therapies for VT. Whether or not more definitive substrate modification with re-vascularization or catheter ablation of VT in select patients may prove an effective means of reducing long-term morbidity and mortality in patients with a history of ES or those at significant risk for future storm awaits further data specifically addressing this topic.

5. Prognosis and clinical implications of ES

While we appear to have adequate pharmacologic and non-pharmacologic measures to help bring an end to the series of arrhythmic events, the mortality associated with these electrical storms is nevertheless very high in carefully analyzed data that include larger numbers of patients with sufficient follow-up. In the AVID trial[12], 34 (38%) of the 90 patients with ES died during follow-up, compared to 15% of those with VT/VF in the absence of ES, and 22% among the remaining patients. Electrical storm was independently associated with a 2.4-fold increase in the risk of death overall (figure 1). Many of the deaths occurred early with a mortality risk that was 5.4-fold higher during the first 3-months following ES (figure 2). [12]

Among patients who received an ICD for primary prevention reasons in MADIT II, those with electrical storm had a 7.4 fold higher risk of death compared to those without treated arrhythmias (figure 1). Once again, early mortality post ES was very prominent, with a 17.8 fold increased risk of death during the first 3 months. Although mortality risk persisted after the initial storm event, this risk was somewhat attenuated, with a relative risk of 3.5 after 3 months (figure 2).[13] Differing from AVID, patients in MADIT II with isolated VT/VF episodes were also at an increased risk of dying with a hazard ratio of 2.5.[12,13] However, patients in MADIT II with ES still had 2.9 fold increased risk of death when compared to those with VT/VF in the absence of ES. Once a patient had a storm event, the mode of death differed from those patients with isolated VT/VF or no arrhythmic events. The rate of non-sudden cardiac death was significantly higher for those with ES (23%) compared to those with isolated VT/VF (8%) and no recorded ventricular arrhythmia (5%). Storm patients were more likely to suffer an ischemic-mediated event (myocardial infarction or angina) as compared to patients without ES. Finally, once storm occurred, the incidence of a recurrent storm episode was 2.3%, 4.7% and 6.2% for years 1, 2 and 3, respectively.[13]

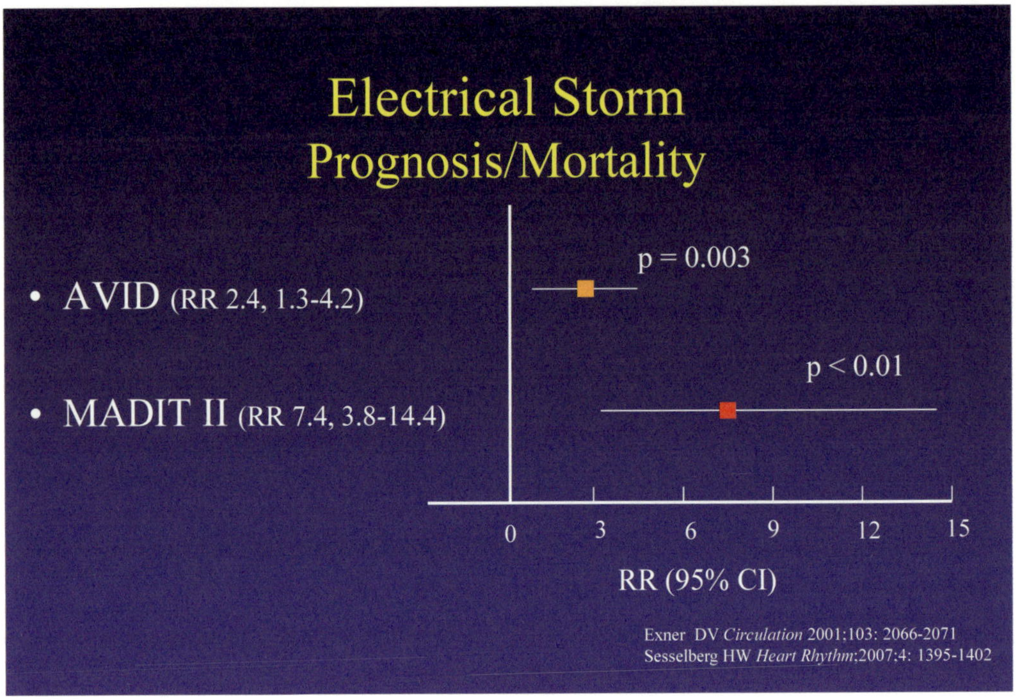
Electrical Storm
Prognosis/Mortality
• AVID (RR 2.4, 1.3-4.2)
• MADIT II (RR 7.4, 3.8-14.4)
p = 0.003
p < 0.01
0
3
6
9
12
15
RR (95% CI)
Exner DV Circulation 2001;103: 2066-2071
Sesselberg HW Heart Rhythm;2007;4: 1395-1402

Fig. 1.

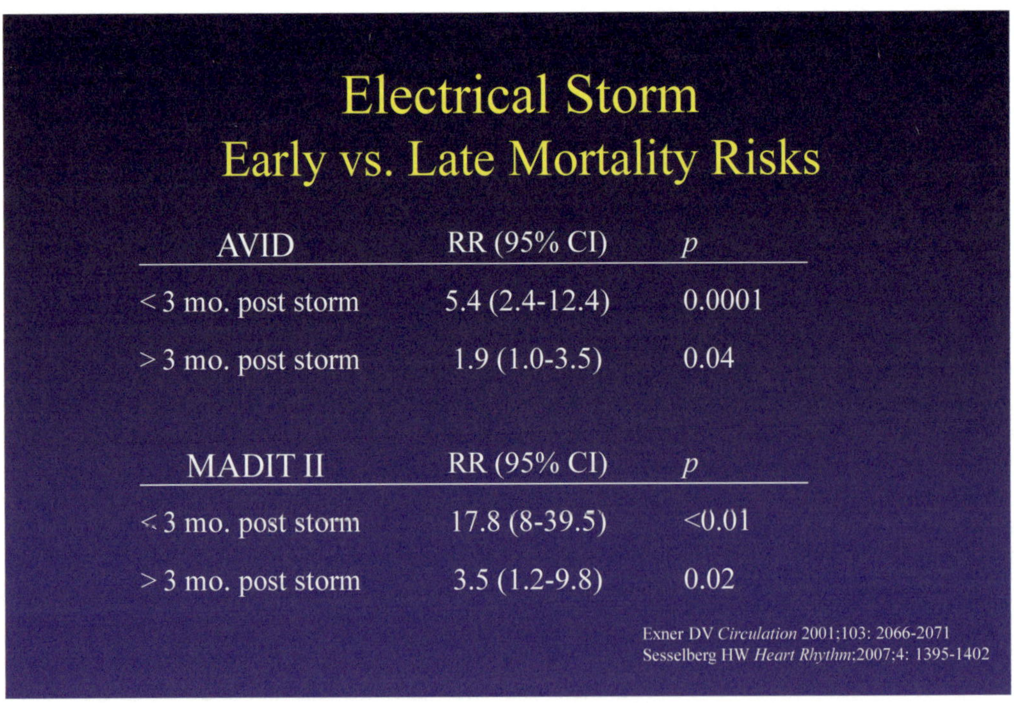
Electrical Storm
Early vs. Late Mortality Risks
AVID RR (95% CI) p
< 3 mo. post storm 5.4 (2.4-12.4) 0.0001
> 3 mo. post storm 1.9 (1.0-3.5) 0.04
MADIT II RR (95% CI) p
< 3 mo. post storm 17.8 (8-39.5) <0.01
> 3 mo. post storm 3.5 (1.2-9.8) 0.02
Exner DV Circulation 2001;103: 2066-2071
Sesselberg HW Heart Rhythm;2007;4: 1395-1402

Fig. 2.

Analysis of these larger trials consistently indicates that in both populations of primary and secondary prevention indications for ICD implant, ES presages mortality, mostly due to non-sudden cardiac causes.[12,13] It is clear that the very immediate mortality associated with ES is not high suggesting that the acute management strategies are relatively successful.[1,2,7,11-21] However, the subsequent mortality is very high and often due to non-arrhythmic causes.[11-13] The initial few months following an episode of electrical storm appear to be a critical window for close monitoring and therapeutic intervention targeting not only the potential arrhythmic causes, but all cardiac issues.[12,13] Whether it is the progressive worsening of the substrate or the additive adverse effects of the armada of medical therapy that these patients are placed on (more likely a combination of these) that is the culprit for the substantially higher mortality is unclear.

The role of the shocks themselves as contributing to myocardial injury and inflammation or even remodeling should not be overlooked. Patients who receive multiple ICD shocks can have detectable troponin elevations consistent with myocardial injury.[1,2,,12, 28,29] Pathological changes including contraction band necrosis, vacuolar cytoplasmic clearing and myocyte loss have been visualized on myocardium under patch electrodes in patients who have experienced multiple defibrillations.[29-31] Myocardial injury or stunning from recurrent defibrillations may activate the neurohormonal cascade responsible for worsening heart failure and ultimately cardiovascular mortality. [1-2,7,11,27, 31-34]

6. Treatment of ES

The treatment of electrical storm entails:

i. Promptly identifying and treating precipitating causes or triggers such as drug toxicities, electrolyte imbalance or acute myocardial ischemia.[1-2,35]

ii. Attempting to understand the underlying cardiovascular substrate for incessant ventricular arrhythmias (ischemia, decompensated heart failure, pause dependent polymorphic VT, etc.).[1,2,35]

iii. Suppressing the ventricular arrhythmias via pharmacologic, device related or interventional mechanisms.[1,2,35]

iv. Establishing a therapeutic regimen with frequent follow-up visits in an effort prevent further ES and mortality in the early vulnerable period.[1-2]

Electrical storm can be a highly-charged clinical situation associated with significant patient anxiety and discomfort, which further elevates sympathetic tone, and leads to an even greater propensity for ventricular arrhythmias.[1-4] The cornerstone of immediate therapy is sympathetic blockade accomplished by the use of intravenous (IV) beta-blocking agents combined with sedatives, usually benzodiazepines.[1-4,7, 22, 35] A beta-one selective agent is often used first, but if ineffective, a nonselective beta-blocker such as propanolol can be substituted. [1,2,35-37] For highly symptomatic patients, intubation and anesthesia may be necessary and even therapeutic.[1-2,38-39] Successful sympathetic manipulation via left stellate ganglionic blockade has been reported in post-myocardial infarction (MI) patients with electrical storm. [40]

In patients with ICDs, device reprogramming may be necessary. Overdrive pacing by increasing the lower rate limit of the ICD may be effective in preventing further electrical storm, particularly when ventricular arrhythmias are pause-dependent or involves tissue automaticity.[1,7,14] While the addition of anti-tachycardia pacing (ATP) will not eliminate the VT trigger, a significant percentage of monomorphic VT can be successfully terminated by

ATP, reducing the anxiety, discomfort and increased sympathetic tone associated with recurrent ICD shocks.[1-2,41] For patients with single chamber defibrillators, consideration can be given to addition of an atrial lead or even upgrade to cardiac resynchronization therapy. These modifications may allow for up-titration of heart failure and anti-arrhythmic therapy. As will be discussed later, in appropriately selected patients, cardiac resynchronization therapy (CRT) with a bi-ventricular implantable cardioverter defibrillator (CRT-D) may reduce the incidence of electrical storm.[42]

The instinct to push anti-arrhythmic agents must be restrained, because with the exception of amiodarone, there is little evidence of benefit and the potential for pro-arrhythmia.[1-,4,7,35] In the absence of significant electrolyte imbalance or drug-induced prolonged QT syndrome with polymorphic VT, amiodarone is often the anti-arrhythmic agent of choice for treatment of ES, with demonstrated benefit in multiple clinical studies.[2,4,6] The efficacy of intravenous amiodarone in ICD patients with storm is also supported by case series.[14,17] If the combination of intravenous amiodarone and beta-blockers does not suppress ES, the addition of lidocaine is sensible.[1,2,14] Certain clinical entities such as electrical storm in the setting of Brugada syndrome are often heart rate sensitive and can be suppressed by using isoproterenol to increase the sinus rate. Isoproterenol infusion has also been used to suppress the VF triggers during electrical storm in patients with Idiopathic VF.[43-44]

Once a patient's arrhythmias have been suppressed, the focus should shift towards evaluation for and treatment of changes in the underlying cardiovascular substrate such as worsening ischemia or heart failure and reduction in left ventricular ejection fraction (LVEF).[1,2,8,12] Larger scale trials have demonstrated that the first few months, post-ES are a critical window for intervention.[1-2,12-13] Diligent implementation and augmentation of therapies with proven mortality benefit in similar patient populations is mandatory. Standard heart failure therapy, particularly beta-blockers should be maximized. Revascularization clearly has a role in preventing sudden cardiac death and reducing the ability to induce ventricular fibrillation and polymorphic ventricular tachycardia. Patients with inducible or spontaneous monomorphic VT do not respond as well to revascularization, likely due to a more scar based substrate rather than direct membrane or channel instability.[45-46] For these patients, aggressive anti-tachycardia pacing should be utilized in an effort to reduce shock burden in the VT zone.[1,2,8,41] The relative benefits and risks of long-term anti-arrhythmic therapy versus catheter ablation of ventricular tachycardia must be weighed. The recently released Substrate Mapping & Ablation in Sinus Rhythm to Halt Ventricular Tachycardia (SMASH-VT) study showed promising results for the ability of substrate mapping to reduce ICD therapy in patients with ischemic cardiomyopathy.[47] However, success rates for catheter ablation for VT can vary based on the substrate and the experience of operators which are factors that need to be taken into consideration (some are difficult to control for). As this promising therapy evolves, it will likely be utilized earlier in the clinical course for patients who receive appropriate ICD therapy.[47-49]

7. Cardiac resynchronization therapy and ES events

Cardiac resynchronization therapy has been reported to halt ES events in some patients and yet it has also been reported to induce ES in others. In patients who present with ES, cardiac resynchronization therapy in a qualified patient, i.e., widened QRS duration, advanced heart failure and depressed left ventricular function, has been shown to resolve the arrhythmic events.[50-52] Paradoxically, there also has been several case reports of ventricular arrhythmia storm post cardiac resynchronization therapy, either de novo implants or upgrades.[53-55] The mechanism of arrhythmia storm has been speculated to be related to the heterogeneous transmural repolarization across the ventricle[56] and possible concealment related to left or bi-ventricular pacing. The programmed pacing from the left ventricular lead of the resynchronization device has been reported to reinitate reentrant ventricular tachyarrhythmias by concealment into a potential VT circuit antidromically setting up conditions allowing for propagation of the wavefront orthodromically within the VT circuit.[57]

It appears that there are specific subsets of patients whose myocardial substrates are more susceptible to proarrhythmic effects related to biventricular pacing. Possibly, premature ventricular contractions (PVC's) that occur during or with biventricular pacing may alter the conduction characteristics and/or the repolarization process sufficiently to set up conditions such as concealment that create sufficient ventricular heterogeneity for arrhythmogenesis. Particular risk factors for these events are as yet unclear and further work is needed for further elucidation. In these patients, it is worthwhile programming the left ventricular pacing off, even if the patient may be pacing dependent. Further intervention can be pursued, whether pharmacologically or non-pharmacologically to modify the substrate. Care providers should also be mindful that the implanted lead(s) may be the culprit serving as the origin for arrhythmia and lead extraction/revision will need to be considered in these cases.

Retrospective data have suggested in a non-randomized population, cardiac resynchronization therapy does not actually result in an overall higher incidence of ventricular arrhythmia storm.[58] These data have limited validity due to it nature of uncontrolled population and varied underlying pathology. The availability of more robust data from randomized clinical trials will be better equipped to address whether or not cardiac resynchronization therapy is actually related to an increased incidence of ventricular arrhythmia storm. The Multicenter Automatic Defibrillator Implantation Trial-Cardiac Resynchronization Therapy (MADIT-CRT) randomized patients with mild congestive heart failure (NYHA Class I-II), LVEF $\leq$30% and widened QRS duration ($\geq$130 msec) to either CRT-D or non-resynchronization ICD device implants. The results from this prospectively randomized trial have not detected an overall proarrhythmic effect related to CRT therapy vs. ICD.[59] In fact, these results reveal patients who are responders to CRT, i.e. patient with improved heart failure status and echocardiographic parameters, experienced a lower incidence of ventricular tachyarrhythmia overall.[60]

8. Ablation therapy for ES events

When electrical storm is persistent or even refractory to drug therapy, catheter ablation should be pursued as appropriate. Ablation strategies utilizing entrainment mapping to identify critical isthmus as well as scar substrate modification have been demonstrated to be effective in reducing arrhythmic events acutely and chronically. Catheter ablation was utilized as an urgent treatment strategy in a study comprising of 95 consecutive patients who presented with recurrent or incessant ventricular arrhythmia and ICD shocks. The patients were already on aggressive antiarrhythmic medical therapy, including 94% on amiodarone. Successful ablation of the ventricular arrhythmia, defined as suppression of any further inducible VT, was achieved in 68 of the 95 patients after more than one ablation procedure. At a median follow-up of 22 months, none of these patients had further ES, and the mortality rate was 9%. In contrast, failure to suppress the clinical VT occurred in 10 of 95 patients and was associated with recurrent ES in all and a 40% rate of cardiac mortality.[61] Catheter ablation success is often defined by the underlying arrhythmic substrate. Catheter ablation may also be effective in reducing drug refractory ES episodes in which VF was repeatedly precipitated by ventricular premature contractions originating from either the left or the right ventricle.[62] However the data for this is not as abundant as the strategy of circuit mapping and elimination of reentrant pathways.

There is now accumulating data that suggest earlier intervention may lead to a higher degree of success. SMASH-VT[47] and the Ventricular Tachycardia Ablation in Addition to Implantable Defibrillators in Coronary Heart Disease (VTACH) trial[63] have shown that early intervention even prior to any clinical ICD appropriate VT therapy can be delayed with successful VT substrate modification by ablation. In a recent study comparing the outcome of patients undergoing VT ablation, a group of patients receiving more appropriate ICD therapy and higher doses of amiodarone prior to successful ablation had a higher risk of further ICD therapy and a need to continue more aggressive medical therapy, as compared with those with less ICD shocks and lower doses of amiodarone needed prior to referral for ablation.[64] Furthermore, there was also a more favorable short-term (1 year) VT-free survival rate in the group being referred for catheter ablation with less advanced arrhythmic conditions. This study included some patients with ES but not all presented with ES.

Elimination of critical isthmuses of most or all potential circuits appears to be important in the suppression of continually inducible ventricular tachycardia and associated with improved patient outcome. This in turn, would logically be related to the extent of underlying myocardial disease. Therefore, the success of the ablation may be, at least in part, linked to the degree of myocardial scarring contributing to the arrhythmic substrate and beyond the technical and knowledge limitations of current ablation procedures. This again stresses the importance of early intervention where the acute success rates for ablation and short-term outcome may be higher. Catheter ablation holds the promise of successful substrate modification in the high-risk patients with ES with short-term outcome in reducing the rates of VT and ICD therapy and yet, data demonstrating an improved patient survival in any randomized fashion is still lacking.[65]

9. Conclusions and future directions

Electrical storm is now a well recognized clinical entity among patients with ICDs. Hopefully with more data based on less heterogeneous ICD populations and with continuing careful scrutiny, we may better understand the precipitating causes and exacerbating factors that lead to these malignant ventricular storms. Of additional importance is that we continue to explore the nature of ICD device programming and the interaction between the type of ICD therapy delivered and future prognosis. Recent data gathered from large ICD populations suggests that the type of therapy delivered ATP vs. ICD shocks may influence future mortality.[66,67] While the occurrence of an electrical storm episode may indicate a changing or worsening cardiovascular substrate, the addition of multiple shock therapies to an already vulnerable cardiovascular milieu could lead to myocardial stunning and further activation of the neurohormonal cascade responsible for adverse electrical and ventricular remodeling. Further research is needed to explore methods to decrease ventricular arrhythmia burden and to delineate appropriate ICD programming for effectively treating ventricular arrhythmias while minimizing the ICD shock burden to patients.

Electrical storm is a critical cardiac condition which demands aggressive intervention. Initial antiarrhythmic therapies need to be followed by a careful and thorough evaluation of the entire cardiac status. With the current treatment armamentarium, immediate mortality can often be averted, but the accompanying high early mortality post-ES calls for aggressive substrate modification aiming at maximized CHF and arrhythmia management as well as reduction of the possible ischemic burden.[7,11,12] Prophylactic measures such as pre-emptive VT substrate modification with ablation or medication hold promise but remain to be established in large series.

10. References

[1] Proietti R, Sagone A. Electrical storm: Incidence, Prognosis and Therapy. Indian Pacing and Electrophysiology Journal 2011;11(2):34-42.

[2] Huang DT, Traub D. Recurrent ventricular arrhythmia storms in the age of implantable cardioverter defibrillator therapy: A comprehensive review. Progress in Cardiovascular Diseases. 2008;51:229-236.

[3] Kowey PR, Levine JH, Herre JM, Pacifico A, Lindsay BD, Plumb VJ, Janosik DL, Kopelman HA, Scheinman MM. Randomized, double-blind comparison of intravenous amiodarone and bretylium in the treatment of patients with recurrent, hemodynamically destabilizing ventricular tachycardia or fibrillation. The Intravenous Amiodarone Multicenter Investigators Group. Circulation 1995;92:3255-63.

[4] Dorian P, Cass D. An overview of the management of electrical storm. Can J Cardiol 1997;13(Suppl A);13A-17A.

[5] Kowey PR. An overview of antiarrhythmic drug management of electrical storm. Can J Cardiol 1996;12(Suppl B):3B-8B.

[6] Credner SC, Klingenheben T, Mauss O, Sticherling C, Hohnloser SH. Electrical storm in patients with transvenous implantable cardioverter-defibrillators: incidence, management and prognostic implications. J Am Coll Cardiol 1998;32:1909-15.

[7] Scheinman MM, Levine JH, Cannom DS, Friehling T, Kopelman HA, Chilson DA, Platia EV, Wilber DJ, Kowey PR. Dose-ranging study of intravenous amiodarone in patients with life-threatening ventricular tachyarrhythmias. The Intravenous Amiodarone Multicenter Investigators Group. Circulation 1995;92:3264-72.

[8] Israel CW, Barold SS. Electrical Storm in patients with an implanted defibrillator: A matter of definition. Annals of Noninvasive Electrocardiology, Volume 12, Number 4, October 2007, pp. 375-382(8).

[9] Myerburg RJ, Castellanos A. Cardiac arrest and sudden cardiac death. In: Zipes DP, Libby P, Bonow RO, et al (eds): Braunwald's Heart Disease: A textbook of cardiovascular medicine. Philadelphia, PA: Elsevier, 2005, p. 865-908.

[10] Wood MA, Ellenbogen KA, Liebovitch LS. Electrical storm in patients with transvenous implantable cardioverter defibrillators. JACC 1999;34:950-51.

[11] Wood MA, Simpson PM, Stambler BS, Herre JM, Bernstein RC, Ellenbogen KA. Long-term temporal patterns of ventricular tachyarrhythmias. Circulation 1995;91:2371-2377.

[12] Exner DV, Pinski SL, Wyse DG, Renfroe EG, Follmann D, Gold M, Beckman KJ, Coromilas J, Lancaster S, Hallstrom AP. Electrical storm presages nonsudden death: the antiarrhythmics versus implantable defibrillators (AVID) trial. Circulation 2001;103:2066-71.

[13] Sesselberg HW, Moss AJ, McNitt S, et al. Ventricular arrhythmia storms in postinfarction patients with implantable defibrillators for primary prevention indications: A MADIT-II substudy. Heart Rhythm 2007; 4:1395-1402.

[14] Gatzoulis KA, Andrikopoulos GK, Apostolopoulos T, Sotiropoulos E, Zervopoulos G, Antoniou J, Brili S, Stefanadis CI. Electrical storm is an independent predictor of adverse long-term outcome in the era of implantable defibrillator therapy. Europace. 2005;7:184-92.

[15] Bänsch D, Bocker D, Brunn J, Weber M, Breithardt G, Block M.Clusters of ventricular tachycardias signify impaired survival in patients with idiopathic dilated cardiomyopathy and implantable cardioverter defibrillators. J Am Coll Cardiol 2000;36:566-73

[16] Stuber T, Eigenmann C, Delacretaz E. Characteristics and relevance of clustering ventricular arrhythmias in defibrillator recipients. Pacing Clin Electrophysiol 2005;28:702-7.

[17] Greene M, Newman D, Geist M, Paquette M, Heng D, Dorian P. Is electrical storm in ICD patients the sign of a dying heart? Outcome of patients with clusters of ventricular tachyarrhythmias. Europace 2000;2:263-9.

[18] Hohnloser SH, Al-Khalidi HR, Pratt CM, Brum JM, Tatla DS, Tchou P, Dorian P. Electrical storm in patients with an implantable defibrillator: incidence, features, and preventive therapy: insights from a randomized trial. Eur Heart J 2006;27:3027-32.

[19] Arya A, Haghoo M, Dehghani MR, et al. Prevalence and predictors of electrical storm in patients with implantable cardioverter-defibrillators. Am J Cardiol 2006;97:389-392.

[20] Verma A, Kilicaslan F, Marrouche NF, Minor S, Khan M, Wazni O, Burkhardt JD, Belden WA, Cummings JE, Abdul-Karim A, Saliba W, Schweikert RA, Tchou PJ, Martin DO, Natale A. Prevalence, predictors, and mortality significance of the causative arrhythmia in patients with electrical storm. J Cardiovasc Electrophysiol 2004;15:1265-70.

[21] Brigadeau F, Kouakam C, Klug D, et al. Clinical predictors and prognostic significance of electrical storm in patients with implantable cardioverter defibrillators. European Heart Journal 2006;27:700-707.

[22] Fries R: Incidence and clinical relevance of short-term recurrent ventricular tachyarrhythmias in patients with implantable cardioverter defibrillator. Int J Cardiol 1997;59:281-4.

[23] Dijkman B, den Dulk K, Wellens HJ. Management of electrical instability after ICD implantation.Pacing Clin Electrophysiol 1995;18:148-51

[24] Kim SG, Ling J, Fisher JD, Wang G, Rameneni A, Roth JA, Ferrick KJ, Gross J, Ben-Zur U, Brodman R. Comparison and frequency of ventricular arrhythmias after defibrillator implantation by thoracotomy versus nonthoracotomy approaches. Am J Cardiol 1994;74:1245-8.

[25] Shukla G, Chaudhry GM, Orlov M. Potential proarrhythmic effect of biventricular pacing: Fact or myth?. Heart Rhythm 2005;2:951-956.
[26] Turitto G and El-Sherif N. Cardiac resynchronization therapy: A review of proarrhythmic and antiarrhythmic mechansisms. Pacing Clin Electrophysiol. 2007;30(1):115-122.
[27] Singh JP, Hall JW, McNitt S, et al. Factors influencing appropriate firing of the implanted defibrillator for ventricular tachycardia/tibrillation: findings from the Multicenter Automatic Defibrillator Implantation Trial II (MADIT-II). J. Am. Coll. Cardiol., Nov 2005; 46: 1712 - 1720.
[28] Hurst TM, Hinrichs M, Breidenbach C, Katz N, Waldecker B. Detection of myocardial injury during transvenous implantation of automatic cardioverter-defibrillators. J Am Coll Cardiol 1999;34:402-8.
[29] Joglar JA, Kessler DJ, Welch PJ, Keffer JH, Jessen ME, Hamdan MH, Page RL. Effects of repeated electrical defibrillations on cardiac troponin I levels. Am J Cardiol 1999;83:270-2.
[30] Singer I, Hutchin GM, Mirowski M, et al. Pathologic findings related to the lead system and repeated defibrillations in patients with the automatic implantable cardioverter-defibrillator. J Am Coll Cardiol 1987;10:382-388.
[31] Epstein AE, Kay N, Plumb VJ. Gross and microscopic pathological changes associated with nonthoracotomy implantable defibrillator leads. Circulation 1998;98:1517-1524.
[32] Poelaert J, Jordaens L, Visser CA, et al. Transesophageal echocardiographic evaluation of ventricular function during transvenous defibrillator implantation. *Acta Anaesthesiol Scand.* 1996;40:913–918.
[33] De Piccoli B, Rigo F, Raviele A, et al. Transesophageal echocardiographic evaluation of the morphologic and hemodynamic cardiac changes during ventricular fibrillation. *J Am Soc Echocardiogr.* 1996;9:71–78.
[34] Runsio M, Bergfeldt L, Brodin LA, et al. Left ventricular function after repeated episodes of ventricular fibrillation and defibrillation assessed by transesophageal echocardiography. *Eur Heart J.* 1997;18:124–131.
[35] Zipes DP, Camm AJ, Borggrefe M, Buxton et al. ACC/AHA/ESC 2006 guidelines for management of patients with ventricular arrhythmias and the prevention of sudden cardiac death: a report of the American College of Cardiology/ American Heart Association Task Force and the European Society of Cardiology Committee for Practice Guidelines (Writing Committee to Develop Guidelines for Management of Patients With Ventricular Arrhythmias and the Prevention of Sudden Cardiac Death). J Am Coll Cardiol 2006;48:e247- e346.
[36] Jordaens LJ, Mekel JM. Electrical storm in the ICD era. Europace 2005;7:181-183.
[37] Tsagalou EP, Kanakakis J, Rokas S, et al. Suppression by propanolol and amiodarone of an electrical storm refractory to metoprolol and amiodarone. Int J Cardiol 2005;99:341-342 Burjorjee JE, Milne B.
[38] Propofol for electrical storm; a case report of cardioversion and suppression of ventricular tachycardia by propofol. *Canadian Journal of Anesthesia* 2002;49:973-977.
[39] Mulpuru SK, Patel DV, Wilbur SL, et al. Electrical storm and termination with propofol therapy: A case report. Int J Cardiol 2007.

[40] Nademanee K, Taylor R, Bailey WE, Rieders DE, Kosar EM. Treating electrical storm: sympathetic blockade versus advanced cardiac life support-guided therapy. Circulation 2000;102:742-7.

[41] Prospective Randomized Multicenter Trial of Empirical Antitachycardia Pacing Versus Shocks for Spontaneous Rapid Ventricular Tachycardia in Patients With Implantable Cardioverter-Defibrillators: Pacing Fast Ventricular Tachycardia Reduces Shock Therapies (PainFREE Rx II) Trial Results Mark S. Wathen, Paul J. DeGroot, Michael O. Sweeney, et al. *Circulation. 2004;110:2591-2596.*

[42] Effect of cardiac resynchronization therapy on the incidence of electrical storm. International Journal of Cardiology. 201;143:330-336.

[43] Isoproterenol as an adjunct for treatment of idiopathic ventricular fibrillation storm in a pregnant woman. Mittadodla PS, Salen PN, Traub DM. Am J Emerg Med. 2010.

[44] Acute and chronic management in patients with Brugada syndrome associated with electrical storm of ventricular fibrillation. Ohgo T, Okamura H, Noda T, Satomi K, Suyama K, Kurita T, Aihara N, Kamakura S, Ohe T, Shimizu W.Heart Rhythm. 2007;6:695-700.

[45] O'Rourke RA. Role of myocardial revascularization in sudden cardiac death. Circulation 1992;85[suppl I]:I112-I117.

[46] Marrouche NF, Verma A, Wazni O, Schweikert R, Martin DO, Saliba W, Kilicaslan F, Cummings J, Burkhardt JD, Bhargava M, Bash D, Brachmann J, Guenther J, Hao S, Beheiry S, Rossillo A, Raviele A, Themistoclakis S, Natale A. Mode of initiation and ablation of ventricular fibrillation storms in patients with ischemic cardiomyopathy. *J Am Coll Cardiol.* 2004; 43: 1715–1720.

[47] Reddy VY, Reynolds MR, Neuzil P, et al. Prophylactic catheter ablation for the prevention of defibrillator therapy. *N Engl J Med* 2007; 357:2657-2665.

[48] Soejima K, Suzuki M, Maisel WH, Brunckhorst CB, Delacretaz E, Blier L, Tung S, Khan H, Stevenson WG. Catheter ablation in patients with multiple and unstable ventricular tachycardias after myocardial infarction: short ablation lines guided by reentry circuit isthmuses and sinus rhythm mapping. *Circulation.* 2001; 104: 664–669.

[49] Mason JW. A comparison of seven antiarrhythmic drugs in patients with ventricular tachyarrhythmias. Electrophysiologic Study versus Electrocardiographic Monitoring Investigators N Engl J Med 1993;329:452-458.

[50] Garrigue S, Barold SS, Hocini M, Jaïs P, Haïssaguerre M, Clementy J. Treatment of drug refractory ventricular tachycardia by biventricular pacing. Pacing Clin Electrophysiol. 2000 Nov;23(11 Pt 1):1700-2.

[51] Nicoletti I, Tomei R, Zanotto G, Dalla Vecchia E, Zorzi E, Vassanelli C. The beneficial effect of biventricular pacing on ventricular tachycardia in a patient with non-ischemic cardiomyopathy. Int J Cardiol. 2008 May 23;126(2):e29-31. Epub 2007 Apr 12.

[52] Tanabe Y, Chinushi M, Washizuka T, Minagawa S, Furushima H, Watanabe H, Hosaka Y, Komura S, Aizawa Y. Suppression of electrical storm by biventricular pacing in a patient with idiopathic dilated cardiomyopathy and ventricular tachycardia. Pacing Clin Electrophysiol. 2003 Jan;26(1 Pt 1):101-2.

[53] Kantharia B, Patel J, Nagra B, Ledley G. Electrical storm of monomorphic ventricular tachycardia after a cardiac-resynchronization-therapy-defibrillator upgrade. Europace 8:8: 625-628.

[54] Bortone A, Macia JC, Leclercq F, Pasquié JL. Monomorphic ventricular tachycardia induced by cardiac resynchronization therapy in patient with severe nonischemic dilated cardiomyopathy. Pacing Clin Electrophysiol. 2006 Mar;29(3):327-30.

[55] Mykytsey A, Maheshwari P, Dhar G, Razminia M, Zheutlin T, Wang T, Kehoe R. Ventricular tachycardia induced by biventricular pacing in patient with severe ischemic cardiomyopathy. J Cardiovasc Electrophysiol. 2005 Jun;16(6):655-8.

[56] Fish JM, Brugada J, Antzelevitch C. Potential proarrhythmic effects of biventricular pacing. J Am Coll Cardiol. 2005 Dec 20;46(12):2340-7.

[57] Reithmann C, Hahnefeld A, Oversohl N, Ulbrich M, Remp T, Steinbeck G. Reinitiation of ventricular macroreentry within the His-Purkinje system by back-up ventricular pacing - a mechanism of ventricular tachycardia storm. Pacing Clin Electrophysiol. 2007 Feb;30(2):225-35.

[58] Nordbeck P, Seidl B, Fey B, Bauer WR, Ritter O. Effect of cardiac resynchronization therapy on the incidence of electrical storm. Int J Cardiol. 2010 Sep 3;143(3):330-6. Epub 2009 Apr 8.

[59] Moss A, Hall W J, Cannom D, Klein H, Brown M, Daubert J, Estes M III, Foster E, Greenberg Henry, Higgins S, Pfeffer M, Solomon S., Wilber D, Zareba W for the MADIT-CRT Trial Investigators. Cardiac-resynchronization therapy for the prevention of heart-failure events. N Engl J Med 2009; 361:1329-1338.

[60] Barsheshet A, Wang PJ, Moss AJ, Solomon SD, Al-Ahmad A, McNitt S, Foster E, Huang DT, Klein HU, Zareba W, Eldar M, Goldenberg I. Reverse remodeling and the risk of ventricular tachyarrhythmias in the MADIT-CRT (Multicenter Automatic Defibrillator Implantation Trial-Cardiac Resynchronization Therapy). J Am Coll Cardiol. 2011 Jun 14;57(24):2416-23.

[61] Carbucicchio C, Santamaria M, Trevisi N, et al. Catheter ablation for the treatment of electrical storm in patients with implantable cardioverterdefibrillators: short- and long-term outcomes in a prospective single-center study. Circulation 2008;117:462-469.

[62] Marrouche NF, Verma A, Wazni O, et al: Mode of initiation and ablation of ventricular fibrillation storms in patients with ischemic cardiomyopathy. J Am Coll Cardiol 43:1715-1720, 2004.

[63] Kuck KH, Schaumann A, Willems S, et al. Catheter ablation of stable ventricular tachycardia before defibrillator implantation in patients with coronary heart disease (VTACH): A multicenter randomized controlled trial. Lancet 2010; 375: 31-40.

[64] Frankel DS, Mountantonakis SE, Robinson MR, Zado ES, Callans DJ, Marchlinski FE. Ventricular Tachycardia Ablation Remains Treatment of Last Resort in Structural Heart Disease: Argument for Earlier Intervention. J Cardiovasc Electrophysiol. 2011 May 3.

[65] Deneke T, Shin DI, Lawo T, Bösche L, Balta O, Anders H, Bünz K, Horlitz M, Grewe PH, Lemke B, Mügge A. Catheter ablation of electrical storm in a collaborative hospital network. Am J Cardiol. 2011 Jul 15;108(2):233-9.

[66] Sweeney MO, Sherfesee L, DeGroot PJ et al. Differences in effects of electrical therapy type for ventricular arrhythmias on mortality in implantable cardivoerter-defibrillator patients. Heart Rhythm. 2010 (7):353-360.

[67] Larsen GK, Evans A, Lambert WE et al. Shocks burden and increased mortality in implantable cardioverter defibrillator patients. Heart Rhythm. 2011; In press.

Part 3

Applications and Clinical Relevance

9

Ventricular Arrhythmias Due to a Transient of Correctable Cause in MADIT-II Patients: Prevalence and Clinical Relevance

Michela Casella et al.*
Cardiac Arrhythmia Research Centre,
Centro Cardiologico Monzino IRCCS, Milan,
Italy

1. Introduction

Post-infarction patients with severe left ventricular dysfunction are at high risk of sudden cardiac death. Antiarrhythmic therapy does not improve survival in such patients and, therefore, implantable cardioverter defibrillators (ICD) emerged as treatment of choice for both primary and secondary prevention of mortality after myocardial infarction (MI). The MADIT (Multicenter Automatic Defibrillator Implantation Trial) (1), and MUSTT (Multicenter Unsustained Tachycardia Trial) trials (2) were the first primary prevention ICD trials documenting a substantial reduction in mortality with an ICD in postinfarction patients with depressed ejection fraction, nonsustained ventricular tachycardia, and inducible sustained ventricular tachycardia. The MADIT II trial broadened the indications for prophylactic ICD use in post-infarction patients with ejection fraction of 30% or less without a requirement for additional risk stratification (3). The benefit from ICD therapy in patients with low ejection fraction was recently confirmed by results from the SCD-HeFT (Sudden Cardiac Death in Heart Failure) (4) and COMPANION (Comparison of Medical Therapy, Pacing, and Defibrillation in Heart Failure) trials (5).

2. Triggers of ventricular arrhythmias

Most investigations failed to reveal a transient cause for the development of ventricular arrhythmias in the majority of patients with severe left ventricular dysfunction. Singh et al. showed that among a comprehensive list of baseline clinical, echocardiographic, and electrophysiological variables in the MADIT-II study, more symptomatic patients (NYHA functional class >II) with blood urea nitrogen (BUN)>25 mg/dl, and no beta-blocker use are

---

* Pasquale Santangeli, Ghaliah Al-Mohani[1], Antonio Dello Russo[1], Francesco Perna[2], Stefano Bartoletti[1], Joseph Gallinghouse, Luigi Di Biase, Andrea Natale and Claudio Tondo[1]
Texas Cardiac Arrhythmia Institute at St David's Medical Center, Austin, TX, USA
[1]*Cardiac Arrhythmia Research Centre, Centro Cardiologico Monzino IRCCS, Milan,*
[2]*Catholic University of the Sacred Heart, Rome,*
Italy

at a higher risk for first appropriate ICD therapy and death (6). Several data suggest that transient triggers (ischemia, heart failure, hypokalemia) may cause such events in a substantial proportion of patients. Ventricular premature Beats (VPB) have been found to trigger ventricular tachycardia (VT) especially in the setting of structural heart disease (7). Psychological stress may also be an important trigger. The impact of sympathetic activity on electrical instability is corroborated by the finding of a decreased baroreflex sensitivity in patients with clinical VT (8,9). In this chapter, we report the prevalence and clinical relevance of ventricular arrhythmias due to a transient arrhythmia triggers in patients with ischemic dilated cardiomyopathy undergoing primary prevention ICD implantation.

3. Methods

We collected data of 31 patients with ischemic cardiomyopathy (age 73±8 years, 25 males) who experienced the first arrhythmic event, defined as appropriate ICD intervention on sustained VT or fibrillation (VF), after the implantation of an ICD according to MADIT-II criteria (i.e. LVEF ≤ 30%). Patients were enrolled in our Institution between 2006 and 2008. All ICDs were uniformly programmed. Stored electrograms and ICD data disks from the included patients were reviewed by two expert electrophysiologists. Episodes of spontaneous sustained VT that were terminated by anti-tachycardia pacing or direct-current cardioversion were identified. VF was defined as a rapid, disorganized rhythm with variable cycle length, morphology, and amplitude of the electrogram with difficulty in precisely identifying all activation complexes. Polymorphic VT was diagnosed when electrograms displayed a ventricular tachycardia with almost constant amplitude but with variability in the cycle length and/or morphology of the electrograms. Monomorphic VT was defined as a ventricular tachycardia with a uniform beat-to-beat cycle length and electrogram morphology.

Transient arrhythmia triggers were assessed at the time of the arrhythmic event by means of a complete clinical and laboratory evaluation, including serum electrolyte assessment, echocardiography and coronary angiography in all patients. Patients whose VT/VF was associated with a transient or correctable cause were classified by two independent and blinded investigators into: acute myocardial ischemic event (including myocardial infarction or unstable angina), proarrhythmic drug reaction, worsening of heart failure, electrolyte imbalance (hypokalemia or hypomagnesemia) or other causes.

Continuous variables are presented as mean ± standard deviation, whereas categorical variables are presented as number and percentages. Comparisons between groups were performed with the two-tailed t test for continuous variables and chi-square test for discrete variables. A probability (p) value <0.05 was considered statistically significant. Analyses were performed with the PASW 18.1 statistical software (SPSS Inc.).

4. Results

Baseline characteristics of the patients included in the study are summarized in Table 1. All patients had ischemic cardiomyopathy and the mean left ventricular ejection fraction was 28% ± 5%. Overall, 19 (61%) patients had ICD shock, either on VT (10/19, 53%) or on VF (9/19, 47%). The remaining 12 (39%) patients experienced effective ATP on VT. The mean time from ICD implantation to the ICD intervention was 23 ± 16 months.

Characteristics	
Total number	31
Age, years	73 ± 8
Sex, males	25 (81)
Age at implant, years	70 ± 8
Type of ICD, n (%)	
Dual-chamber	25 (81)
Single-chamber	6 (19)
Sinus Rhythm, n (%)	23 (74)
Atrial Fibrillation, n (%)	8 (26)
Risk factors, n (%)	
Smoke	6 (19)
Hypertension	8 (26)
Diabetes	10 (32)
Hypercholesterolemia	12 (39)
Drug Therapy, n (%)	
Beta blockers	30 (97)
ACE-Inhibitors	31 (100)
Diuretics	17 (55)
Statins	28 (90)
Left ventricular EF, %	28 ± 5
NYHA functional class	2.4 ± 0.7
Creatinine, mg/dL	1.4 ± 0.4

Table 1. Baseline clinical characteristics of the study patients.

The mean time from ICD implantation to the first arrhythmic event was 24±16 months. The first arrhythmic event consisted of VF in 9 (29%) and sustained VT in 22 (71%) patients, of which 10 treated with an ICD shock and 12 with effective anti-tachycardia pacing. No significant differences in baseline characteristics were found between patients with different types of ICD intervention. A transient or correctable trigger for the arrhythmic event was identifiable in 9 (29%) patients and consisted of worsening heart failure in 5 (16%), clinical and angiographic evidence of acute ischemia in 3 (10%) and electrolyte abnormalities (i.e. hypokalemia) in 1 (3%). Ventricular fibrillation was more often associated with a transient trigger compared with sustained VT (67% vs. 14%, respectively, p=0.007). Interestingly, all three patients with acute ischemia as a trigger had VF as arrhythmic event.

5. Discussion

A number of well-known precipitating factors significantly increase the electrical instability of the heart. Among them, exacerbation of heart failure is one of the most important trigger factor suggesting that arrhythmia may simply be a marker of already-worsening HF. In our study worsening heart failure constituted 16% of cases. Previous analysis of the SCD-HeFT data (10) showed findings similar to those of the MADIT-II study. In the SCD-HeFT study, 33% of HF patients received an ICD shock, and among those patients, the most common cause of death was progressive HF (10,11). Myocardial ischemia is important factor. In this study, there were three patients in whom myocardial ischemia was proven to be the trigger for electrical instability and presented with VF as arrhythmic event. VF and myocardial ischemia are inseparable. Presence of one precipitates and perpetuates the other. Transmural heterogeneities in myocardial action potential and ionic currents produce transmural asymmetry in conduction during acute ischemia. Acute transmural ischemia depresses the excitability and velocity of conduction more rapidly in the epicardium than in the endocardium leading to increased dispersion. The occurrence of potentially lethal arrhythmia is the end result of a cascade of pathophysiological abnormalities (12-14). Other triggering factors include the development of electrolyte disturbances such as profound hypokalemia, which was demonstrated in one of our patients. Electrical instability is enhanced upon patients in whom drug treatment for congestive heart failure often acts to further increase electrolyte disturbances.

6. Clinical implication

The ICD has become the therapy of first choice to prevent sudden cardiac death in high-risk patients. Our study also supports the well-understood clinical notion that continued clinical vigilance toward preventing heart failure exacerbations and coronary events might decrease the risk of sudden cardiac death and ICD therapy in these patients. Interestingly importance of heart failure deterioration (i.e.,worsening of clinical status) suggests that this subset of patients have a wider margin to deteriorate and have additional predictive value as a determinant of ICD therapy. This also supports the evidence that in sicker heart failure subjects, the cause of death is more likely owing to pump failure. These results are corroborated by recent studies that show that preventing progression of heart failure with cardiac resynchronization therapy reduces the incidence of arrhythmic events (15,16).

Acute myocardial ischemia in high risk patients is arrhythmogenic, often leading to fatal outcome in the clinical setting. The arrhythmic outcome of an event between trigger and substrate differs. Genetic predisposition and governing responses of ion channels to myocardial ischemia might have a greater role than what is known at present. Efforts to understand these arrhythmias better can do early identification of patients with myocardial ischemia prone to arrhythmias. One of the most important aspects of the current study relates to potential prognostic implications of triggers. At present, there is a paucity of information on this clinically important issue.

Finally, in interpreting our results, it must be recognized that not all triggers causing arrhythmias appropriate ICD shocks for VT/VF would have been detected, and further identification of clinical triggers may help us to higher surveillance and vigilance of possible triggers to avoid primary shock that further deteriorate mortality and heart failure progression, increase in sympathetic tone that may give rise to proarrhythmic side effects of antiarrhythmic drugs may also constitute a precipitating factor for recurrent ventricular tachycardia or fibrillation.

7. Conclusion

Due to the increasing number of patients with severe left ventricular dysfunction, further studies are needed to optimize priority of such patients for ICD therapy. Optimal pharmacologic and anti-ischemic (CABG, percutaneous transluminal coronary angioplasty) therapy, accurate and rapid correction of electrolytes disturbances are essential for proper prevention of shock and mortality in addition to ICD therapy.

8. References

[1] Moss AJ, Hall WJ, Cannom DS, et al.: Improved survival with an implanted defibrillator in patients with coronary disease at high risk for ventricular arrhythmia. Multicenter Automatic Defibrillator Implantation Trial Investigators. N Engl J Med 1996, 335:1933–1940.

[2] Buxton AE, Lee KL, Fisher JD, et al.: A randomized study of the prevention of sudden death in patients with coronary artery disease. Multicenter Unsustained Tachycardia Trial Investigators. N Engl J Med 1999, 341:1882–1890.

[3] Moss AJ, Zareba W, Hall WJ, et al.: The Multicenter Automatic Defibrillator Implantation Trial II Investigators. Prophylactic implantation of a defibrillator in patients with myocardial infarction and reduced ejection fraction. N Engl J Med 2002, 346:877–883.

[4] Sudden Cardiac Death in Heart Failure Trial: (SDC-HeFT). Available at: http://www.sicr.org. Accessed July 26, 2004. Recent (as yet unpublished) study finalizing debate regarding usage of amiodarone for primary prevention of mortality in postinfarction patients with low EF and providing evidence for a beneficial effect of ICD therapy in both ischemic and nonischemic cardiomyopathy patients.

[5] Bristow MR, Saxon LA, Boehmer J, et al.: Cardiac-resynchronization therapy with or without an implantable defibrillator in advanced chronic heart failure. N Engl J Med 2004, 350:2140–2150.

[6] C. Israel and S. Barold, Electrical storm in patients with an implanted defibrillator: a matter of definition, Ann Noninvas Electrocardiogr 12 (2007), pp. 375–382.

[7] Rosman J, Hanon S, Shapiro M, Evans SJ, Schweitzer P. Triggers of sustained monomorphic ventricular tachycardia differ among patients with varying etiologies of left ventricular dysfunction. Ann Noninvasive Electrocardiol 11: 113-117, 2006.

[8] Credner SC, Klingenheben T, Mauss O, et al. Electrical storm in patients with transvenous implantable cardioverter-defibrillators: Incidence, management and prognostic implications. J Am Coll Cardiol 1998;32:1909–1915.

[9] Nademanee K, Taylor R, Bailey WE, et al. Treating electrical storm: Sympathetic blockade versus advanced cardiac life support-guided therapy. Circulation 2000;102:742–747.

[10] Poole JE, Johnson GW, Hellkamp AS, et al. Prognostic importance of defibrillator shocks in patients with heart failure. N Engl J Med 2008;359:1009 –17.

[11] Moss AJ, Greenberg H, Case RB, et al. Long-term clinical course of patients after termination of ventricular tachyarrhythmia by an implanted defibrillator. Circulation 2004;110:3760 –5.
[12] Janse MJ, Wit AL. Electrophysiological mechanisms of ventricular arrhythmias resulting from myocardial ischemia and infarction. Phys Rev 1989;69:1049–169.
[13] Carmeliet E. Cardiac ionic currents and acute ischemia: from channels to arrhythmias. Phys Rev 1999;79:917–1017.
[14] Casciol WE, Johnson TA, Gettes LS. Electrophysiologic changes in ischemic ventricular myocardium: I. Influence of ionic, metabolic and energetic changes. J Cardiovasc Electrophysiol 1995;l6:1039–62.
[15] Higgins SL, Hummel JD, Niazi IK, et al. Cardiac resynchronization therapy for the treatment of heart failure in patients with intraventricular conduction delay and malignant ventricular tachyarrhythmias. J Am Coll Cardiol 2003;42:1454 –9.
[16] Bristow MR, Saxon LA, Boehmer J, et al. Cardiac-resynchronization therapy with or without an implantable defibrillator in advanced chronic heart failure. N Engl J Med 2004;350:2140 –50.

10

ICDs in Clinical Trials: Assessment of the Effects of Omega-3 Polyunsaturated Fatty Acids from Fish Oils on Ventricular Tachycardia and Ventricular Fibrillation

A. Mirrahimi[1,3], L. Chiavaroli[1,3], K. Srichaikul[1,3], J.L. Sievenpiper[1,5], C.W.C. Kendall[1,3,6] and D.J.A. Jenkins[1,2,3,4]

[1]*Clinical Nutrition & Risk Factor Modification Center*

[2]*Department of Medicine, Division of Endocrinology and Metabolism, St Michael's Hospital, Toronto, Ontario*

[3]*Department of Nutritional Sciences*

[4]*Department of Medicine, Faculty of Medicine, University of Toronto, Toronto, Ontario*

[5]*Department of Pathology and Molecular Medicine, Faculty of Health Sciences, McMaster University, Hamilton, Ontario*

[6]*College of Pharmacy and Nutrition, University of Saskatchewan, Saskatoon, Saskatchewan*

Canada

1. Introduction

In its most recent assessment, the American Heart Association (AHA) estimated that in the United States alone there were 5.8 million people with heart failure (HF) in 2006 (Lloyd-Jones, Adams et al. 2010). HF is further estimated to be affecting 23 million people worldwide (McMurray, Petrie et al. 1998). Sudden cardiac death (SCD) is the cause of 28-68% of all mortalities in heart failure patients, the majority of which is due to ventricular tachycardia (VT) or ventricular fibrillation (VF) (Engelstein ED 1998). Implanted cardioverter-defibrillators (ICDs) have been used for nearly 30 years to effectively stop VT or VF, thereby significantly improving sudden cardiac arrhythmic death outcomes in high risk patients (DiMarco 2003). Despite the major success of ICDs, implanted patients continue to experience VT and VF episodes and a range of possible side effects that make it desirable to use ICDs only in situations where necessary.

Anti-arrhythmic drugs are used to reduce the frequency of ventricular arrhythmias in patients with frequent ICD shock. They reduce the ventricular rate of VT so that there is better hemodynamic tolerance and more responsiveness to termination by anti-tachycardia pacing or low energy cardioversion. These drugs also suppress other arrhythmias that cause symptoms or interfere with ICD function and cause "inappropriate" shocks (which may occur in up to 29 percent of ICD patients with substantial impact on their quality of life) (Knilans and Prystowsky 1992; Steinberg, Martins et al. 2001). These "inappropriate" shocks are caused by a variety of arrhythmias including sinus tachycardia, atrial fibrillation, and nonsustained ventricular tachycardia (Pacifico, Hohnloser et al. 1999; Nanthakumar, Paquette et al. 2000). However, anti-arrhythmic drugs are not always well tolerated.

Ultimately, ICD patients are expected to have further arrhythmic episodes and experience ICD shocks which, along with the risks of discharge and “inappropriate” shock, can significantly and adversely affect the patients’ quality of life. Therefore, it is essential to find ways to prevent recurrent episodes of arrhythmias that lead to VT and VF.

Since the first observation of low risk of cardiac death in the study of Greenland Eskimos (Kromann and Green 1980) with high intakes of Omega-3 polyunsaturated fats (PUFAs) from sea mammals and fish, Omega-3 PUFAs have been suggested to have potential beneficial anti-arrhythmic properties (Burr, Fehily et al. 1989; Armstrong, Wieland et al. 1994) and hence have been considered for the treatment of high risk patients with arrhythmias (especially those at immediate risk, i.e. VT/VF patients). ICD patients, are high risk individuals and have been of particular interest in clinical trials investigating the effects of PUFAs on ventricular arrhythmias. Because ICDs are capable of terminating arrhythmias and recording their occurrence and their specific types, the risk of mortality is greatly reduced and the end point which might have resulted in death is averted. Therefore, such studies also have the potential to allow for a crossover design (Leaf, Albert et al. 2005; Raitt, Connor et al. 2005; Brouwer, Zock et al. 2006).

But, are Omega-3 PUFAs an appropriate, effective, and sustainable treatment for averting VT and VF?

Randomized controlled trials in ICD patients have produced powerful and illuminating data regarding the role of this dietary supplement and could potentially have much to offer for other dietary and lifestyle intervention trials.

2. Ventricular fibrillation and fish

Sustained ventricular arrhythmias, which include VT and VF, are the most common cause of sudden cardiac death (SCD) and are hence considered the most relevant endpoint in regards to the harder SCD endpoint when assessing their occurrence using ICDs (Engelstein ED 1998).

Over the last 6 years, 3 double-blind, placebo controlled, randomized studies have been published that used fish oils in patients with ICDs to observe time to first ventricular arrhythmia event post ICD implantation (Leaf, Albert et al. 2005; Raitt, Connor et al. 2005; Brouwer, Zock et al. 2006). None of these trials successfully demonstrated whether or not Omega-3 PUFA supplementation has any preventive effects in ICD patients. These studies were first summarized in a meta-analysis by Jenkins et al. (Figure 1) in which they showed a small non-significant overall effect with a relative risk of 0.93 [95% CI, 0.70-1.24] when comparing the incidence of first ICD discharge in Omega-3 PUFA supplementation versus the placebo (Jenkins, Josse et al. 2008).

Another meta-analysis in the following year confirmed the original findings of Jenkins et al. Bouwer et al. showed a non-significant beneficial effect from fish oil in terms of ventricular tachyarrhythmias or death when compared to a placebo (Hazard ratio (HR) of 0.90 [95% CI; 0.67-1.22]) (Brouwer, Raitt et al. 2009). In their sub group analyses, Brouwer and colleagues showed that the potential beneficial role of fish oils in ventricular arrhythmias was non-significant across all subject types: the HR for fish oils vs. placebo in patients with an

Study Name	No. of Events / No. of Participants: Fish Oil	Control	Relative Risk (95% CI)	Weight, %
Leaf et al., 2005	57/200	78/202	0.74 (0.56-0.98)	33.12
Raitt et al., 2006	51/100	41/100	1.24 (0.92-1.69)	31.33
Brouwer et al., 2005	81/273	90/273	0.90 (0.70-1.15)	35.55
Overall	I^2=67.9%		0.93 (0.70-1.24) P= 0.63	100.00

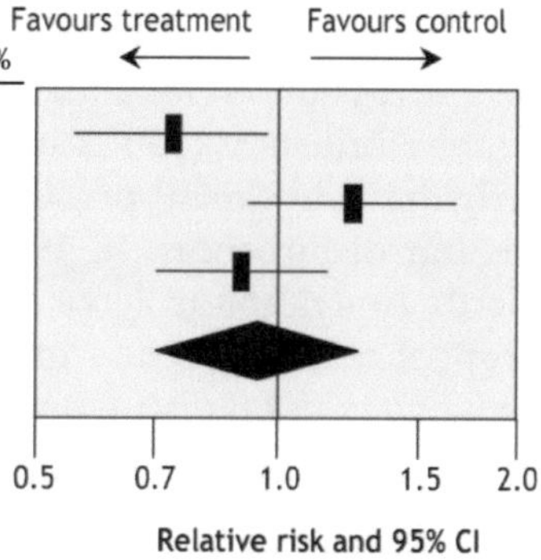

Fig. 1. Meta-analysis of implantable cardioverter defibrillator discharge in studies of fish-oil supplementation. Adapted from Jenkins et al., CMAJ 2008 (Jenkins, Josse et al. 2008).

ejection fraction (EF) ≤30 was 0.80 [95% CI 0.58-1.12]. In patients with established coronary artery disease at baseline, the HR was 0.79 [95% CI 0.6-1.06]. Lastly, in patients with an EF>30 the risk was actually increased, though not significantly, with an HR of 1.18 [95% CI 0.64-2.18].

Moreover, with further data available to them as the original authors of two of the published studies (Brouwer and Raitt); they were also able to pool their data to perform more subgroup analyses that showed a range of deleterious outcomes in various subject types (Figure 2). Most notably, Brouwer et al. showed significantly higher risk of ventricular tachyarrhythmia in patients who used fish oils and were also on lipid-lowering medications with an adjusted HR of 1.48 [95% CI 1.01-2.18].

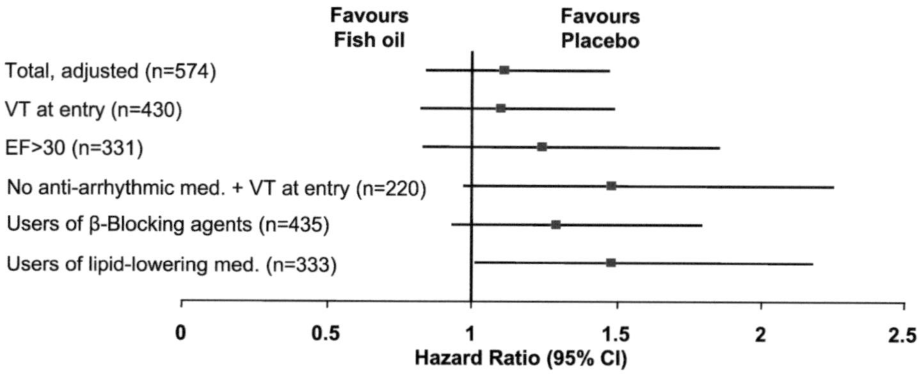

Fig. 2. Hazard ratios of fish oil treatment for time to first ventricular tachyarrhythmia in the pooled analyses (Raitt, Connor et al. 2005; Brouwer, Zock et al. 2006) in the entire study population (primary analysis) and subgroups (subgroup analyses). Adjustments were made for age, gender, ejection fraction, smoking status, New York Heart Association class for angina pectoris, New York Heart Association class for dyspnoea, valvular heart disease, prior myocardial infarction, cardiomyopathy, ventricular tachycardia as index arrhythmia, ventricular fibrillation as index arrhythmia, and use of anti-arrhythmic medication at baseline. Adapted from: Brouwer et al., European Heart Journal 2009 (Brouwer, Raitt et al. 2009).

3. Atrial fibrillation and fish

Although VT and VF are the major concerns with regards to ICD patients, they are not the only arrhythmias; for long considered a benign and inconsequential type of arrhythmia, Atrial Fibrillation (AF) is now becoming a large concern globally. It is the most common arrhythmia in clinical practice, resulting in approximately 1/3 of admissions due to cardiac rhythm disturbances. In 1996/1997 alone, the ATRIA investigators estimated 2.3 million North Americans to have AF (Go, Hylek et al. 2001). Friberg et al. also illustrated that hospital admissions due to AF increased 66% between the late 1970s and late 1990s and continue to rise (Friberg, Buch et al. 2003).

More recently, AF has also been implicated as an independent predictor of VT/VF incidence in ICD patients. Stein et al. showed that ICD patients with AF had a multi-variate adjusted HR of 1.89 [95% CI 1.33-2.69] for VT/VF occurrence in the first year after implantation (Stein, Mittal et al. 2009). Similar findings were also produced by other previous trials, including the PROFIT and the 'JEWEL-AF-study' (Stein, Euler et al. 2002; Klein, Lissel et al. 2006).

Fish oils have therefore been proposed as effective in the treatment and prevention of AF. It is hypothesized that Omega-3 PUFAs preserve normal electrophysiological function (Richardson, Iaizzo et al. 2011). Despite postulated mechanisms, a recent meta-analysis suggests that there is much heterogeneity in the current literature and complexity of AF pathology. Therefore, these PUFAs require further studies prior to solidly claiming their place as a potential therapy. Liu et al. demonstrated that Omega-3 PUFA intake was not significantly associated with a reduction in AF episodes (an odds ratio (OR) of 0.81 [95%CI, 0.57-1.15] for AF incidence) in patients with established heart disease, such as those who have had a coronary artery bypass graft (CABG), persistent AF, or open heart surgery (Liu, Korantzopoulos et al. 2011). In an editorial in the same publication (Liu, Korantzopoulos et al. 2011), Drs. Ramadeen and Dorian elaborated on the reasons why this meta-analysis did not show the anticipated outcomes that were observed in the animal studies (Ramadeen and Dorian 2011; Richardson, Iaizzo et al. 2011). Dorian et al. discussed the mechanisms by which Omega-3 PUFAs can be potentially beneficial may not in fact be due to their antiarrhythmic properties (Ramadeen and Dorian 2011) which in other trials have also been questioned since in some, Omega-3 PUFAs showed pro-arrhythmic activity (Raitt, Connor et al. 2005), but rather due to preventing structural remodelling and fibrosis through their anti-inflammatory properties (Ramadeen, Laurent et al. 2010; Saravanan, Davidson et al. 2010). However, for Omega-3 PUFAs to have any potential efficacy in patients with arrhythmias, their use must be established long before the disease progresses into longer episodes of AF (persistent and permanent). Thus, those with existing heart disease may experience no benefit.

4. Fish oils as the solution

It can be said with absolute certainty that the collapse of our fish stocks due to overfishing is inevitable at the current rate of consumption. Global catches have been declining since the late 1980s (Figure 3A) (Watson and Pauly 2001), and the number of collapsed stocks has been increasing exponentially since 1950 (Figure 3B) (Worm, Barbier et al. 2006; Costello, Gaines et al. 2008). The number and rate of extinctions of marine populations have increased catastrophically and will continue. When projected forward these data indicate a complete collapse of commercially exploited stocks by 2050 (Pauly, Alder et al. 2003; Worm, Barbier et al. 2006).

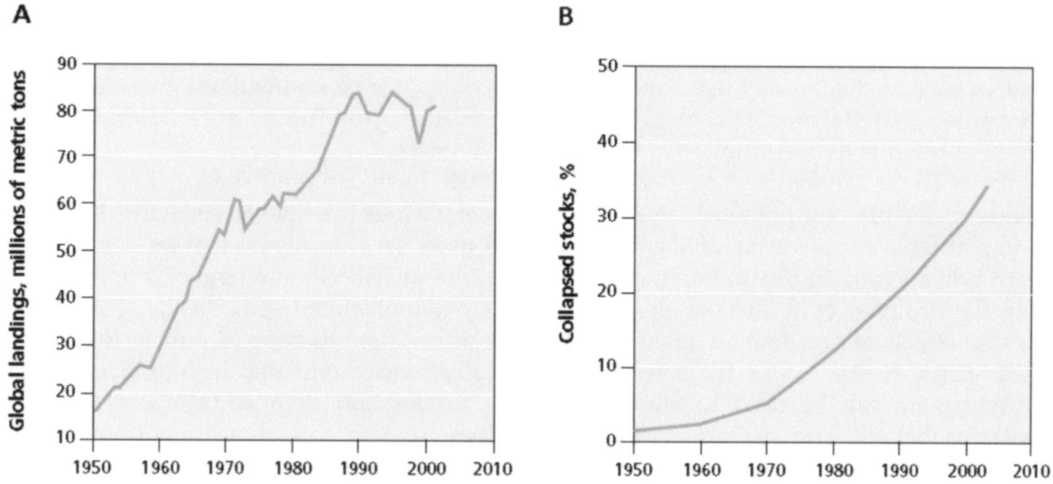

Fig. 3. Global Fishery Trends. (A) Global catch trends from 1950 to 2000, corrected for overreporting by China (Watson and Pauly 2001). (B) Stock collapse: Decline to 10% of their respective historic maximum yield in fish whose stocks have been exploited (n < 10 000; in 64 large marine ecosystems) (RFAD-2007; Worm, Barbier et al. 2006; Costello, Gaines et al. 2008). Adopted from Jenkins et al., CMAJ 2009 (Jenkins, Sievenpiper et al. 2009).

The current data on ICD patients in the three trials summarized first by the Jenkins et al. meta-analysis in 2008 and further investigated by the Brouwer et al. meta-analysis in 2009, certainly ascertains the uncertainty of the benefits of fish oils in this population of patients with heart disease (Jenkins, Josse et al. 2008; Brouwer, Raitt et al. 2009). Brower et al., further elaborates on the potential harms of Omega-3 PUFAs from fish in this population of ICD users, from the population of the combined studies of Raitt et al. and Brouwer et al. (Raitt, Connor et al. 2005; Brouwer, Zock et al. 2006; Brouwer, Raitt et al. 2009).

In regards to fish oil benefits for AF prevention, studies show variable results and are overall inconclusive (Liu, Korantzopoulos et al. 2011). Despite the proposed 2.5-fold increase by 2050 in AF prevalence (Go, Hylek et al. 2001), the lack of certainty on the therapeutic role of fish oils contrasts with the certainty that increased fish consumption will simply shorten the survival of fish stocks with little or no human health benefit. Therefore, continuing to advocate fish consumption to confer health benefits may at present be inappropriate.

5. Conclusion

In conclusion, Omega-3 PUFAs may have some potential beneficial effects in heart disease, likely not because of having potential anti-arrhythmic effects, as was long postulated, but possibly through their anti-inflammatory properties that may in the long term prevent structural remodelling, and damage to the electrical conduction pathways of the myocardium provided it is initiated before structural remodelling begins (Ramadeen and Dorian 2011). However, Omega-3 PUFAs have not been shown to be effective in ICD studies and may possibly be harmful in preventing VT/VF episodes after remodelling and fibrosis has occurred (Liu, Korantzopoulos et al. 2011; Jenkins, Josse et al. 2008; Brouwer, Raitt et al. 2009).

To gamble the existence of our planet's fish stocks (Jenkins, Sievenpiper et al. 2009) on inconclusive data instead of using lifestyle modifications and appropriate pharmaceutical treatments, that can be as beneficial, is not responsible, both for patients and planetary health. It is therefore important to consider the use of other sustainable sources of Omega-3 PUFAs, such as the recently developed algal sources by Martek and DuPont pharmaceutical companies (Arterburn, Oken et al. 2008; Surette 2008), for future exploration of their potential benefits in heart disease as well as other diseases.

Lastly, ICDs in randomized controlled clinical trials have certainly shown their merit in assessing the different potential benefits or harms of various treatments, since the discharge of implantable cardioverter defibrillators can be used as a surrogate marker for sudden death while avoiding death. For example, in the case of fish oils the larger compiled data from the Brouwer et al. meta-analysis quite clearly demonstrated some of the unexpected harmful effects of high fish oil intake in ICD patients on statin therapy (Brouwer, Raitt et al. 2009). Ergo, future larger trials with other detailed measurements, including diet and lifestyle data, can be used to assess further outcomes and help address controversial questions that will form the basis of future guidelines.

6. Disclosure

Arash Mirrahimi, Korbua Srichaikul have no conflicts of interest.

Laura Chiavaroli holds a casual Clinical Research Coordinator position at Glycemic Index Laboratories, Toronto, CANADA.

John L Sievenpiper has received several unrestricted travel grants to present research at meetings and one unrestricted research grant from The Coca-Cola Company. He has also received travel funding and honoraria from Archer Daniels Midland and International Life Sciences Institute (ILSI) North America; and research support, consultant fees, and travel funding from Pulse Canada.

Cyril WC Kendall has received honoraria or travel funding from the Canola Council of Canada, Pulse Canada, the Saskatchewan Pulse Growers, the Almond Board of California, the International Tree Nut Council Nutrition Research & Education Foundation, Loblaws, Barilla, and Unilever; has been on the speakers' panel for the Almond Board of California and the International Tree Nut Council; and has received research grants from the Canola Council of Canada, Pulse Canada, the Saskatchewan Pulse Growers, Agriculture and Agri-Food Canada, Loblaws, Unilever, Barilla, the Almond Board of California and the International Tree Nut Council.

David JA Jenkins has served on the scientific advisory board for or received research support, consultant fees, or honoraria from Griffin Hospital in New Haven for the development of the NuVal System, Abbott Laboratories, Procter and Gamble Technical Centre Limited, Kellogg's, Quaker Oats Canada, Barilla, Solae, Unilever, Hain Celestial, Loblaws Inc., The Coca Cola Sugar Advisory Board, Nutritional Fundamentals for Health, Sanitarium Company, Herbalife International, Pacific Health Laboratories Inc., Science Advisory Council Agrifoods and Agriculture Canada, Canadian Agriculture Policy Institute (CAPI), Soy Advisory Board - Dean Foods, Partners with Glycemic Index Laboratories, Metagenics/MetaProteomics, Bayer Consumer Care, Oldways Preservation Trust, The Almond Board of California, The California Strawberry Commission, Orafti, the Canola and Flax Councils of Canada, Pulse Canada, and the Saskatchewan Pulse Growers. David JA Jenkins also holds additional grant support from the CIHR, Canadian Foundation for Innovation (CFI), Ontario Research Fund (ORF), and Advanced Foods and material Network (AFMNet), International Tree Nut Council Nutrition Research and Education Foundation and the Peanut Institute, and Alpro Soy Foundation.

7. References

Armstrong, V. W., E. Wieland, et al. (1994). "Serum antibodies to oxidised low-density lipoprotein in pre-eclampsia and coronary heart disease." *Lancet* 343(8912): 1570.

Arterburn, L. M., H. A. Oken, et al. (2008). "Algal-oil capsules and cooked salmon: nutritionally equivalent sources of docosahexaenoic acid." *J Am Diet Assoc* 108(7): 1204-9.

Brouwer, I. A., M. H. Raitt, et al. (2009). "Effect of fish oil on ventricular tachyarrhythmia in three studies in patients with implantable cardioverter defibrillators." *Eur Heart J* 30(7): 820-6.

Brouwer, I. A., P. L. Zock, et al. (2006). "Effect of fish oil on ventricular tachyarrhythmia and death in patients with implantable cardioverter defibrillators: the Study on Omega-3 Fatty Acids and Ventricular Arrhythmia (SOFA) randomized trial." *JAMA* 295(22): 2613-9.

Burr, M. L., A. M. Fehily, et al. (1989). "Effects of changes in fat, fish, and fibre intakes on death and myocardial reinfarction: diet and reinfarction trial (DART)." *Lancet* 2(8666): 757-61.

Costello, C., S. D. Gaines, et al. (2008). "Can catch shares prevent fisheries collapse?" *Science* 321(5896): 1678-81.

DiMarco, J. P. (2003). "Implantable cardioverter-defibrillators." *N Engl J Med* 349(19): 1836-47.

Engelstein ED, Z. D. (1998). "Sudden cardiac death. In: Alexander RW, Schlant RC. Fuster V, editors. Hurst's the heart. 9th ed. New York: McGraw Hill, 1998:1081-112."

Friberg, J., P. Buch, et al. (2003). "Rising rates of hospital admissions for atrial fibrillation." *Epidemiology* 14(6): 666-72.

Go, A. S., E. M. Hylek, et al. (2001). "Prevalence of diagnosed atrial fibrillation in adults: national implications for rhythm management and stroke prevention: the AnTicoagulation and Risk Factors in Atrial Fibrillation (ATRIA) Study." *JAMA* 285(18): 2370-5.

Jenkins, D. J., A. R. Josse, et al. (2008). "Fish-oil supplementation in patients with implantable cardioverter defibrillators: a meta-analysis." *CMAJ* 178(2): 157-64.

Jenkins, D. J., J. L. Sievenpiper, et al. (2009). "Are dietary recommendations for the use of fish oils sustainable?" *CMAJ* 180(6): 633-7.

Klein, G., C. Lissel, et al. (2006). "Predictors of VT/VF-occurrence in ICD patients: results from the PROFIT-Study." *Europace* 8(8): 618-24.

Knilans, T. K. and E. N. Prystowsky (1992). "Antiarrhythmic drug therapy in the management of cardiac arrest survivors." *Circulation* 85(1 Suppl): I118-24.

Kromann, N. and A. Green (1980). "Epidemiological studies in the Upernavik district, Greenland. Incidence of some chronic diseases 1950-1974." *Acta Med Scand* 208(5): 401-6.

Leaf, A., C. M. Albert, et al. (2005). "Prevention of fatal arrhythmias in high-risk subjects by fish oil n-3 fatty acid intake." *Circulation* 112(18): 2762-8.

Liu, T., P. Korantzopoulos, et al. "Prevention of atrial fibrillation with omega-3 fatty acids: a meta-analysis of randomised clinical trials." *Heart* 97(13): 1034-40.

Lloyd-Jones, D., R. J. Adams, et al. "Heart disease and stroke statistics--2010 update: a report from the American Heart Association." *Circulation* 121(7): e46-e215.

McMurray, J. J., M. C. Petrie, et al. (1998). "Clinical epidemiology of heart failure: public and private health burden." *Eur Heart J* 19 Suppl P: P9-16.

Nanthakumar, K., M. Paquette, et al. (2000). "Inappropriate therapy from atrial fibrillation and sinus tachycardia in automated implantable cardioverter defibrillators." *Am Heart J* 139(5): 797-803.

Pacifico, A., S. H. Hohnloser, et al. (1999). "Prevention of implantable-defibrillator shocks by treatment with sotalol. d,l-Sotalol Implantable Cardioverter-Defibrillator Study Group." *N Engl J Med* 340(24): 1855-62.

Pauly, D., J. Alder, et al. (2003). "The future for fisheries." *Science* 302(5649): 1359-61.

Raitt, M. H., W. E. Connor, et al. (2005). "Fish oil supplementation and risk of ventricular tachycardia and ventricular fibrillation in patients with implantable defibrillators: a randomized controlled trial." *JAMA* 293(23): 2884-91.

Ramadeen, A. and P. Dorian "Omega-3 polyunsaturated fatty acids: food or medicine?" *Heart* 97(13): 1032-3.

Ramadeen, A., G. Laurent, et al. "n-3 Polyunsaturated fatty acids alter expression of fibrotic and hypertrophic genes in a dog model of atrial cardiomyopathy." *Heart Rhythm* 7(4): 520-8.

RFAD-2007 "Rome (Italy): Fisheries and Aquaculture Department, The state of world fisheries and aquaculture 2006" Food and Agriculture Organization of the United Nations (2007).

Richardson, E. S., P. A. Iaizzo, et al. "Electrophysiological mechanisms of the anti-arrhythmic effects of omega-3 fatty acids." *J Cardiovasc Transl Res* 4(1): 42-52.

Saravanan, P., N. C. Davidson, et al. "Cardiovascular effects of marine omega-3 fatty acids." *Lancet* 376(9740): 540-50.

Stein, K. M., D. E. Euler, et al. (2002). "Do atrial tachyarrhythmias beget ventricular tachyarrhythmias in defibrillator recipients?" *J Am Coll Cardiol* 40(2): 335-40.

Stein, K. M., S. Mittal, et al. (2009). "Predictors of early mortality in implantable cardioverter-defibrillator recipients." *Europace* 11(6): 734-40.

Steinberg, J. S., J. Martins, et al. (2001). "Antiarrhythmic drug use in the implantable defibrillator arm of the Antiarrhythmics Versus Implantable Defibrillators (AVID) Study." *Am Heart J* 142(3): 520-9.

Surette, M. E. (2008). "The science behind dietary omega-3 fatty acids." CMAJ 178(2): 177-80.

Watson, R. and D. Pauly (2001). "Systematic distortions in world fisheries catch trends." *Nature* 414(6863): 534-6.

Worm, B., E. B. Barbier, et al. (2006). "Impacts of biodiversity loss on ocean ecosystem services." *Science* 314(5800): 787-90.

11

Application of the Bispectral Index (BIS) During Deep Sedation for Patients with ICD Testing

Małgorzata Kuc[1], Maciej Kempa[2], Magdalena A.Wujtewicz[1], Radosław Owczuk[1] and Maria Wujtewicz[1]
[1]*Department of Anesthesiology and Intensive Care*
[2]*II Department of Cardiology and Electrotherapy of the Heart*
Medical University of Gdańsk,
Poland

1. Introduction

Epidemiological studies indicate that in Europe, sudden cardiac death (SCD) is the cause of from 20 to 159 deaths per 100 thousand inhabitants / year. In the United States, therefore, die each year from 300 to 400 thousand people. Unfortunately, as shown by the results of clinical trials, the use of antiarrhythmic drugs doesn't protect the majority of patients before the onset of malignant ventricular arrhythmias which are the main cause of SCD.

Other methods of treatment aimed at eliminating the causes of arrhythmia, such as antiarrhythmic cardiosurgery or transvenous ablation of arrhythmias can be effectively used only in a narrow group of patients.

Thus, the treatment of choice in treating people at risk of SCD became the implantation of cardioverter-defibrillator (ICD). The creator of the idea of this method of treatment was Mieczyslaw (Michel) Mirowski (1924-1990). In the sixties of the last century, he started work on the design of devices capable of cardiac rhythm track, and in case of serious ventricular arrhythmias automatically restore sinus rhythm.

The first implantation of automatic defibrillators (without cardioversion) occurred in the Johns Hopkins Hospital in Baltimore in 1980.

Evaluation of the effectiveness of the ICD in SCD preventing has been the subject of many studies. Based on the results, the indications for ICD implantation can be divided into secondary prevention, for patients after cardiac arrest with ventricular fibrillation (VF) or a previous episode settled ventricular tachycardia (VT) and the primary prevention, including patients without malignant arrhythmias.

Immediately after ICD implantation, and after 3-7 days you need to confirm the correct positioning of defibrillation electrodes. This allows you to confirm the correct location and accuracy of programming. While the study conducted a few days after ICD implantation should confirm the effectiveness of the algorithm of therapy chosen by the proper detection of induced control ventricular fibrillation. There are two methods to identify and then a safety margin between defibrillation pulse energy of the programmed and actual energy required to terminate VF. These are: a test to verify the effectiveness of defibrillation and defibrillation threshold measurement.

Verification test is relatively simple and involves initiation of ventricular fibrillation (with special functions ICD) and the interruption of the arrhythmia using a defibrillation pulse of a certain energy. This energy has to be correspondingly smaller (usually about half) than the maximum available under the ICD model so as to provide sufficient (double) safety margin taking into account possible fluctuations in defibrillation threshold in the future. After a successful test, defibrillation energy in the ICD is programmed at the highest available value.

Defibrillation threshold (DFT) is the lowest energy allows to interrupt of VF. Measurement of DFT requires several times causing arrhythmia, and then interrupting by the pulse of different energy power. The usual method of DFT testing is protocol of gradually reduced defibrillation energy. The test is typically commenced from the defibrillation pulse energy of 15-20 J. After each successful defibrillation is performed the next, using a pulse of energy usually lower about 10-20%. In this way, determines the highest energy, with which the successive VF is not interrupted. Another way of determining the DFT is to use the protocol with gradually increases defibrillation energy. In this case, the testing deffibrillation pulse has the energy gradually increased (10-20%), ranging from 5-8 J until the determination of the lowest value allowing interrupt VF.

The most commonly used algorithms of VF induction are the two:

1. High-speed "burst-type" stimulation - depending on the model of ICD, shock for ventricular pacing pulse energy of several volts and frequencies of 30-50 Hz for a few to tens seconds (Fig. 1)
2. "Shock on T" method - triggering the ICD pulse of energy from 0.5 J to a few J at the top of the T wave (Fig. 2)

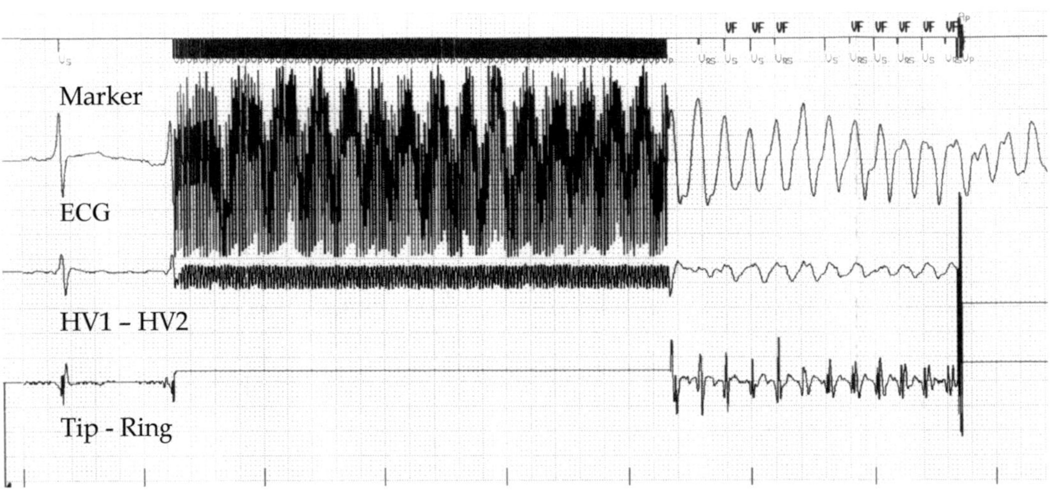

Fig. 1. An example of initiation of ventricular fibrillation by "burst-type" stimulation. Record of the Biotronik 1000 TMS programmer. Implantable cardioverter-defibrillator Belos VR - Biotronik. Paper travel 25 mm / sec.

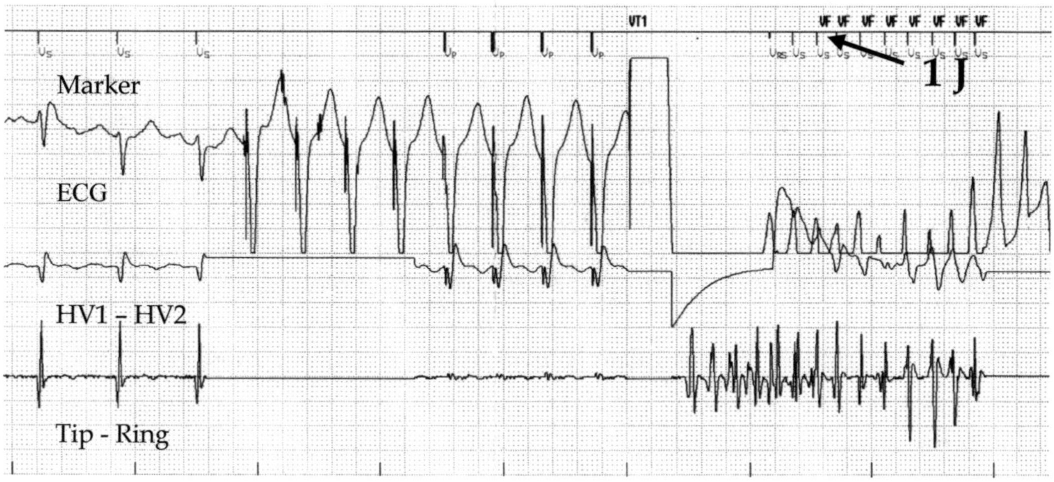

Fig. 2. An example of initiation of ventricular fibrillation by "shock on T " method. Record of the Biotronik 1000 TMS programmer. Implantable cardioverter-defibrillator Belos VR - Biotronik. Paper travel 25 mm / sec.

In some patients, repeated attempts to induce VF using both methods didn't cause arrhythmia.[1] Then you need to induction of VF by stimulation of burst-type beam pulses from the ICD connected with simultaneous induction of unsynchronised impulse from an external defibrillator.[2,3] This method is sometimes called as a "shock,on burst".[4]

1.1 Indications for ICD implantation

The subject of many randomized controlled trials was to establish a factor to identify patients at risk of SCD. Because coronary artery disease is the basis of ventricular arrhythmias in 80% of cases and cardiomiopathies (especially dilated cardiomiopathy) in 15%, that is why these diseases were a major subject of study in clinical trials of primary prevention.

Although coronary heart disease and dilated cardiomyopathy are the most common cause of ventricular arrhythmias, European Society of Cardiology guidelines allow implantation of the ICD in primary prevention in patients with less recognizable diseases. An example is hypertrophic cardiomyopathy (HCM) with the associated additional risk factors such as syncope, family history, left ventricular wall thickness of over 30 mm, abnormal pressure response during exercise and paroxysmal ventricular tachycardia (Indications class IIa / C). Patients with HCM and episodes of ventricular fibrillation or ventricular tachycardia should undergo ICD implantation in secondary prevention.

In the course of arrhythmogenic right ventricular cardiomyopathy, ICD in primary prevention can be used in patients with syncope of unknown etiology or in the case of family history, and when the disease process coverage also includes the left ventricle (Indications class IIa/C)

Also, a genetic disease such as long QT syndrome (LQTS), a polymorphic ventricular tachycardia-dependent catecholamine or Brugada syndrome may be the indication for prophylactic ICD implantation. In the case of LQTS, ICD can be implanted for primary prevention in patients with recurrent syncope despite beta-blocker therapy (Indications class IIa /B) or those without syncope but with known types of LQT2 and LQT3 treated as being particularly strongly associated with risk of SCD (Indications class IIb/B). Patients with Brugada syndrome with characteristic changes in the resting ECG, recurrent syncope, as well as those with polymorphic ventricular tachycardia dependent on catecholamines and syncope, may also be secured in the ICD in primary prevention (Indications class IIa /C).

2. Indications for ICD implantation in primary prevention (Chart 1)

Definitely relate to more potential patients than secondary prevention (Existing guidelines of the European Society of Cardiology)

a. Prior myocardial infarction (after more than 40 days after MI)
   1. NYHA II or III, EF ≤ 35%, the expected survival time exceeds one year. (Indication class I/A)
   2. NYHA I, EF ≤ 30-35%, the expected survival time exceeds one year. (Indications Class IIa /B)

b. Dilated cardiomyopathy noncoronarogenes
   1. NYHA II or III, EF ≤ 35% of the expected survival time exceeds one year. (Indication class I/B)
   2. NYHA I, EF ≤ 30-35%, the expected survival time exceeds one year. (Indications class IIb /C)

c. Cardiomyopathy, whatever the reasons (coronary and noncoronary)

NYHA III and IV, EF ≤ 35%, the duration of the QRS complex > 120 msec is recommended ICD implantation with the function resynchronisation stimulation (Indications Class I/A).

3. Indications for ICD implantation in secondary prevention

1. Past cardiac arrest caused by ventricular tachyarrhythmias in the mechanism irreversible or unknown.
2. Ventricular tachycardia leading to unconsciousness.
3. Syncope of unknown etiology, in patients in whom in electrophysiological examination there was haemodynamically not tolerated VT or VF.

4. Cause of reversible and irreversible of cardiac arrest

The cause is reversible, such as ventricular fibrillation, which occurred in the course of acute ischemia, myocardial infarction or acute phase of myocarditis is not an indication for ICD implantation, but the underlying disease requires treatment of any subsequent verification of indications.

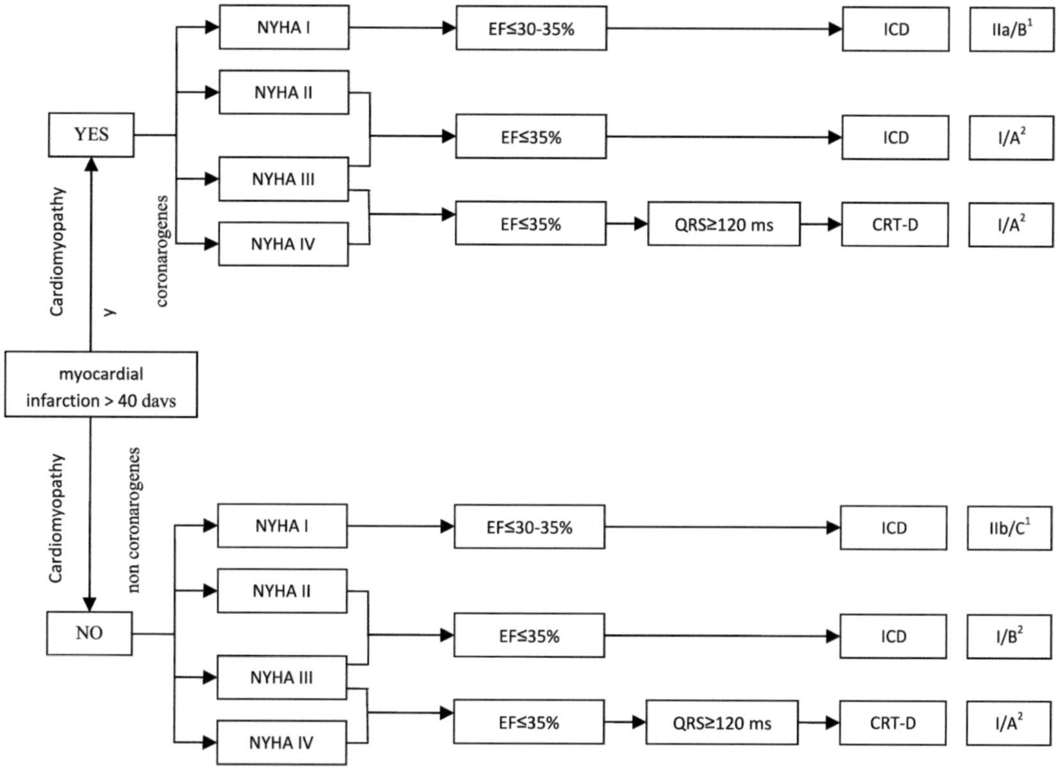

(1) According to ACC / AHA / ESC 2006 guidelines for management of patients with ventricular arrhythmias and the prevention of sudden cardiac death[5].

(2) According to ESC Guidelines for the diagnosis and treatment of acute and chronic heart failure 2008[6].

Chart 1. Indications for ICD implantation for primary prevention of SCD.

The cause is irreversible, eg electrolyte abnormalities associated with cardiac arrest or an adverse impact pharmacotherapy consisting of induction of arrhythmias. Irreversibility in these situations is the result of inability to confirm that any of these factors have been isolated and not accompanied to any other cause leading to arrhythmia. Furthermore, it's no possible to prevent with 100% certainty a recurrence of the situation. Thus, experts agree that in their current situation to propose ICD implantation for patient.

5. Anesthesia for ICD patients

ICD implantation is used in heavily loaded cases (see - the indications for implantation). Their ejection fraction (EF) is often reduced to 10-15%. Therefore, the anesthetic drugs used and their dosage must be carefully chosen. At the same time dose must be sufficient to run the entire test of the defibrillator. Can not be allowed to shallow sedation or anesthesia.

In the Medical University of Gdansk, ICD is implanted since 1995. Initially, the ICD was implanted under general anesthesia. Prolonged surgery and prolonged anesthesia deteriorating general condition of patients. Since 1999, the ICD is implanted under local anesthesia and deep sedation is performed to verify the proper functioning of the ICD and to determine the defibrillation threshold.

6. Preparing the patient for deep sedation

Patients presenting to the ICD implantation are being prepared for surgery by cardiologists. After determining cardiac indications, patients are evaluated in the ASA & NYHA scales. Due to the burden that is the heart muscle disease and often accompanies circulation failure, patients should be anesthetized by an experienced anesthesiologist. Before the procedure, EF is evaluated in ECHO-cardiography. In the operating room is used hemodynamic monitoring and oxygen therapy. It is advisable to monitor the depth of anesthesia because the ICD test is performed 2 - 4 times to set the parameters of defibrillation and monitoring its effectiveness. The interval between the performance of subsequent tests claims of at least 2 - 3 minutes. You can't afford to have shallowing of anesthesia. Anesthesia or deep sedation to the ICD test have to be short. Initiation of ventricular fibrillation isn't a painful process. Therefore, in this type of anesthesia isn't used painkillers.

7. Hypnotics used to the ICD test

1. Etomidate (marketed as Amidate by *Labeler*)- carboxyl derivative of imidazole. Its anesthetic effect is a consequence of the depressant effects on the brain stem reticular creation, through stimulation of GABA. After etomidate injection some patients may appear myoclonus and dyskinesia. Etomidate causes luxury perfusion the heart muscle. Oxygen consumption by the myocardium under the influence of etomidate doesn't change, while the coronary circulation increases by 20%. This action is preferable to a thiopental actions on the myocardium, which also increases coronary blood flow but may also increase oxygen consumption by the myocardium. Etomidate doesn't affect heart rate, slightly decreases peripheral resistance, which increases cardiac output. Onset of action after 15 - 45 sec. Duration of action 3 - 12 min.
2. Sodium thiopental - (marketed as thiopental by Biochemie) - thiobarbiturate soluble in lipids. Its anesthetic effect is inhibiting formations in the brain stem reticular. The drug rapidly decreases blood pressure but slow injection causes compensatory mechanisms, and this decline is poorly defined. This drug has a beneficial effect on peripheral vascular resistance, because it increases slightly due to a compensatory increase in sympathetic activity. Heart rate after administration of thiopental is usually increased. . Thiopental exerts a direct negative inotropic effect on the myocardium. Reduces stroke volume. Onset of action after 20 sec. Duration of action 5 - 10 min.
3. Propofol (marketed as Diprivan by Astra Zeneca) is a derivative of phenol. Changes in heart rate are less pronounced than after thiopental. Often, however, patients taking beta - blockers are observed bradycardia. Propofol causes hypotension, which is causing a negative inotropic effect and a decrease in peripheral resistance. Onset of action after 15 - 45 sec. Duration of action 5 - 10 min.
4. Midazolam (marketed as Dormicum by Roche) - a water-soluble derivative of benzodiazepine. The action arises upon binding the drug to benzodiazepine receptors which enhance the inhibitory effect of GABA on the transfer of stimulus. The action of midazolam on the cardiovascular system is poorly expressed. Heart rate does not change or slightly increases. Myocardial contractility decreases slightly. Oxygen

consumption by heart muscle and blood flow don't change. Onset of action after 30 - 60 sec. Duration of action 15 - 30 min.

8. Monitoring depth of sedation

1. EEG (Narcotrend) - this device is an attempt to automatic analysis of EEG. Induction of anesthesia is characterized by a decrease of frequency and amplitude of EEG waves. With deepening anesthesia theta waves appear. Delta waves are characteristic of deep anesthesia. The next stage is the occurrence of burst supression until the abolition of the electrical activity of the brain characterized by the occurrence of isoelectric line.
2. BIS - bispectral index - includes data of bispectral and conventional EEG analysis. Unites the different EEG parameters into a whole by presenting the average value of diversified parameters of bioelectrical activity of the brain. BIS is an absolute number from 0 to 100, where 100 represents the state of vigilance, and 0 is an electric silence (tab.1). With values of BIS from 83 to 89 amnesia occurs, and with values from 64 to 72 - loss of consciousness.

BIS 100	the standby, preserved the memory
BIS 65- 80	sedation
BIS 40 – 65	moderate to profound loss of consciousness with amnesia recommended for general anesthesia
BIS < 40	coma

Table 1. The interpretation of the BIS value.

3. AEP - auditory evoked potentials - assess the electrical activity of the brain caused by an acoustic stimulus. The severity of the waves depends on the state of consciousness. The smallest is asleep. The patient before anesthesia is placed in the ear headphones, which emit a loud signal. The patient's skin as opposed to the measure by BIS should be prepared. Abrasive tape rubs calluses, as to produce a skin reaction in the form of browning.
4. Entropy of EEG - (Datex Ohmeda Entropy). Evaluation of depth of anesthesia consists of an analysis of two parameters: ST-state entropy - the value characteristic for the brain's electrical activity - EEG and RE - response entropy - includes EEG and electromyography of facial muscles. During deep anesthesia, these values didn't differ. Unexpected increase in RE in relation to the SE may be a sign of inadequate anesthesia.

Among these depth of sedation monitoring techniques, least time-consuming and the simplest for interpretation is the BIS. Enhanced monitoring of patients for testing the ICD provides a good opportunity to assess the quality of anesthesia, while you carefully assess the condition of patients wake up after surgery. This monitoring is particularly important in patients at increased risk of general anesthesia.

9. A study comparing etomidate, sodium thiopental and propofol[7]

From the data presented in the literature shows that thiopental and propofol should be used in people with heart disease with caution. On the other hand, studies conducted in patients treated with electrotherapy because of arrhythmia, demonstrated safety of these anesthetics[8,9,10].We resigned from the use of etomidate because of the substantial degree of severe myoclonus which persisted even after waking patients, which is observed by Pacifico et al[11].Before our study thiopental and propofol was used in smaller doses (3 mg / kg and 1 mg / kg). Such proceedings require additional doses of medication between validation tests of the defibrillator-cardioverter. Determination of the dose of sodium thiopental 5 mg / kg and propofol 1.5 mg / kg allowed testing the ICD after a single dose in most patients. This has created a comfortable environment for staff and patients. Increasing the dose of drugs wasn't accompanied by an increased incidence of side effects such as apnea or prolonged time to recovery of full consciousness.

The study group comprised 50 patients in whom anesthesia was performed using propofol (27 patients) or thiopental (23 patients). Ejection Fraction (EF) was assessed before the treatment by echocardiography. Patients weren't premedication. Monitoring of the patient in the operating room included ECG, blood pressure by the indirect method, pulse oximetry and bispectral index (BIS). In the operating room was used passive oxygen therapy by mask with oxygen flow 6 l / min. Anesthesia for this procedure was intravenous anesthesia without intubation. For anesthesia was administered a single dose of propofol (1.5 mg/kg) or sodium thiopental (5 mg/kg) during 30 sec. Evaluation of the parameters was started after the administration of hypnotics.Statistical analysis was performed using Statistica 7.1 PL (StatSoft, Tulsa, USA).The results, depending on the nature of their distribution, verified by test W (Shapiro and Wilk) , presented as arithmetic mean (standard deviation) or median (range). To compare the data with normal distribution and comparable variances (Levene's test verification) was used T-test for independent variables, in the absence of homogeneity of variance was used T-test with separate variance estimation (Welch test). In cases of non-normality of variables, the comparison test was used Mann-Whitney test. Relationships between variables were tested using the R-Spearman's test of rank correlation. Adopted for significant p-value $p<0.05$.

10. Results

The results are shown in Table 2.

Parameter	Thiopental		Propofol		p
	Median	Range	Median	Range	
EF (%)	30	15–75	40	15–70	0,55
Loss of ciliary reflex (sec)	51	27-83	55	20-240	0,45
Ciliary reflex recovery time (sec)	315	123–776	440	214-660	0,0099
BIS output	98	94-99	98	89 -98	0,47
BIS minimum	38	23–76	42	32 -82	0,05
BIS minimum - time after the administration of medicines	93	50-312	140	54-570	0,04
BIS after waking	75	59-84	72	59-89	0,74
SpO_2 output	98	96–100	98	95-100	0,17
final SpO_2	98	97-100	98	95-100	0,9
Time from wake up to return to baseline BIS (sec)	397	181-841	253	122–549	0,0004
Final BIS	98	94–99	98	89-98	0,47

Table 2. Results of the variables studied.

EF ranged from 15 to 75% in both groups. The average age in both groups did not differ significantly. There was no difference in the disappearance of ciliary reflex in both groups (fig. 3), but its disappearance followed later in patients treated with propofol than in patients treated with thiopental (fig 4).

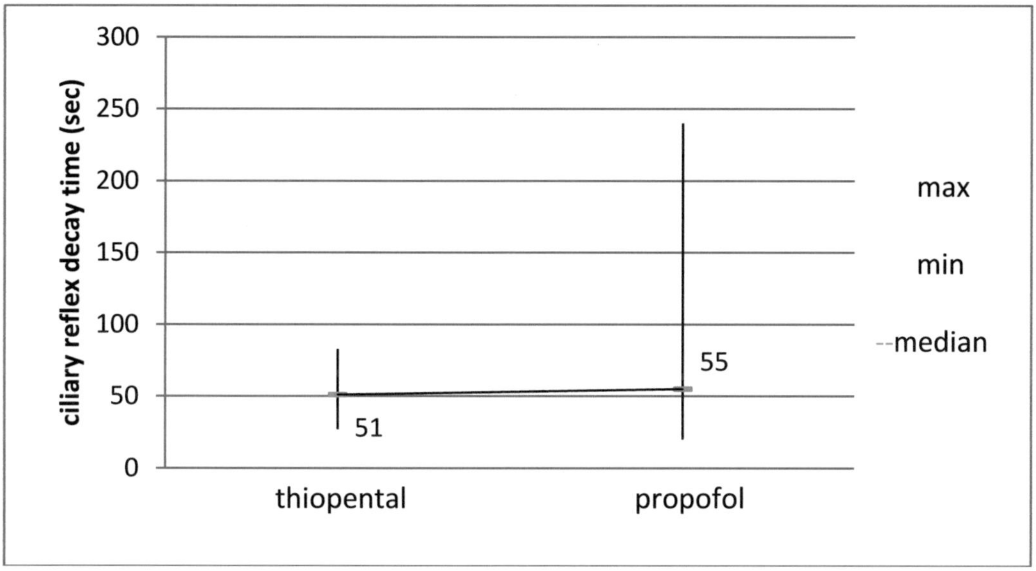

Fig. 3. Ciliary reflex decay time (sec).

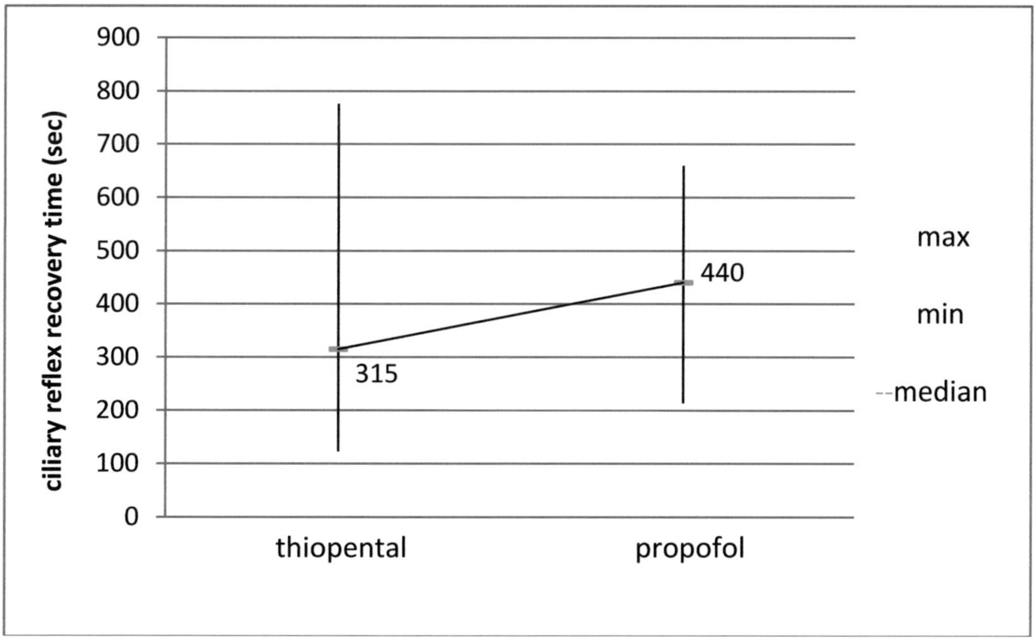

Fig. 4. Ciliary reflex recovery time (sec).

Output BIS values in both groups were identical. There was a significant statistical difference in the minimal BIS value, and the time, in which the minimal BIS was achieved. Minimum BIS values were lower in patients receiving thiopental than in patients receiving propofol (fig 5).

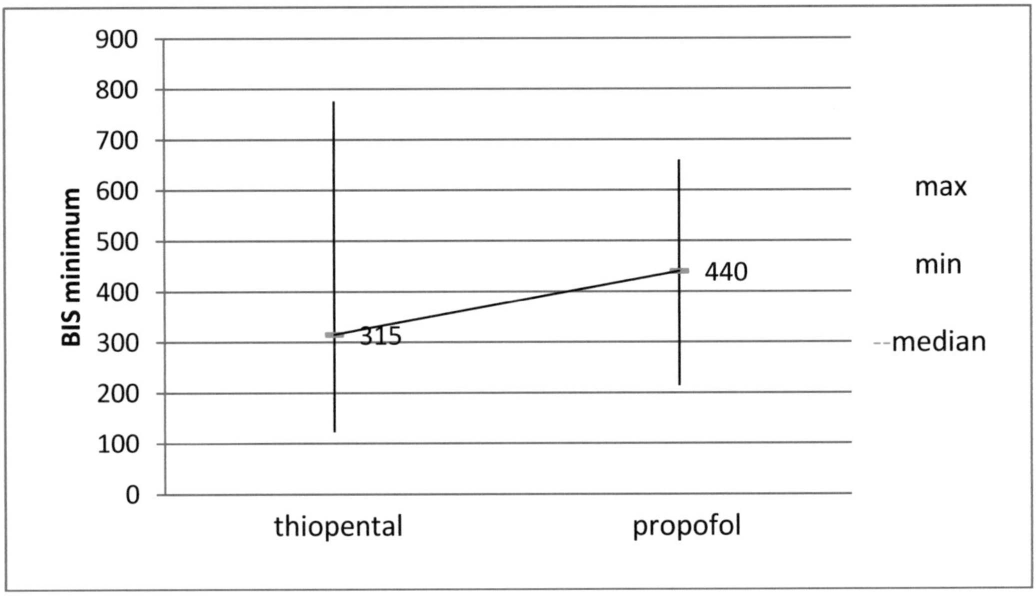

Fig. 5. BIS minimum.

BIS value at which managed to make verbal-logical contact with the patients were comparable in both groups (72 in patients receiving thiopental and 73 in patients receiving propofol). Only the time of return to baseline BIS, was differed in both groups. It was significantly shorter in patients receiving propofol than in patients receiving thiopental (fig. 6).

11. Discussion

Implantable cardioverter defibrillators are implanted under general anesthesia [12,13,14] or under local anesthesia [11,15]. Schematic procedure depends on the experience and standards of conduct [7]. For short-term cardiac procedures are recommended short-acting drugs, without the depressive effects on the cardiovascular system [11-15]. Clinical research comparing effects of etomidate, propofol and sodium thiopental, used for anesthetic during cardiac procedures didn't show any hemodynamic differences in these patients [8,9,10]. Data from the literature shows that sodium thiopental and propofol should be used in people with heart disease with caution. On the other hand, studies in patients treated with electrotherapy because of arrhythmia, demonstrated safety of these anesthetics [8,9,10].

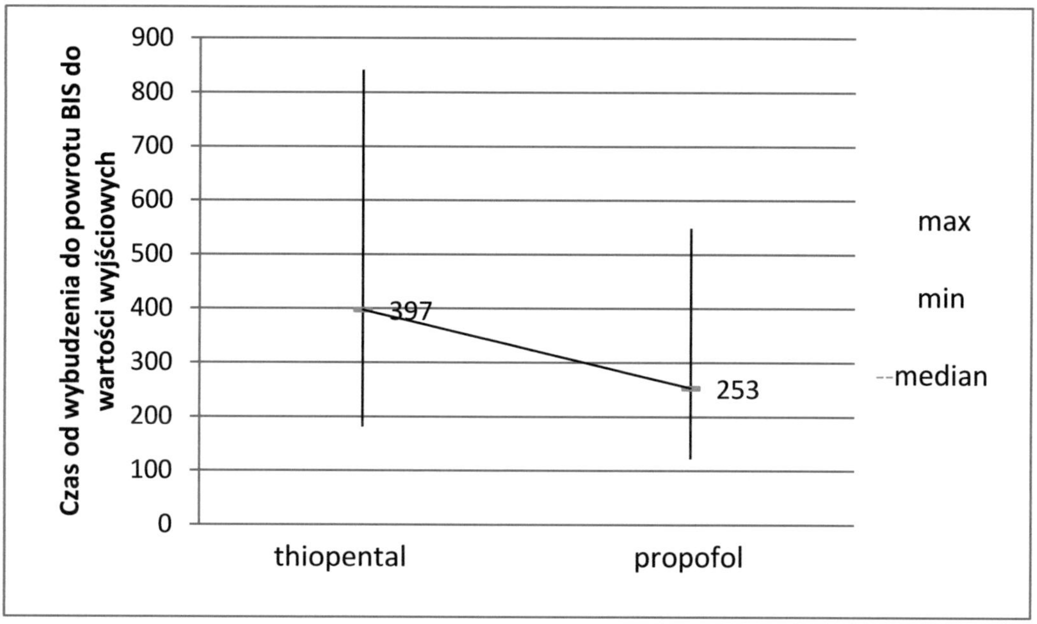

Fig. 6. Time of the return of baseline BIS.

During anesthesia, there was no reduction in oxygen saturation in patients receiving propofol and in patients receiving sodium thiopental. Monitoring depth of anesthesia was performed using the BIS [16]. The study of quality of sedation was made based on its evaluation. [16]. In our study we observed that BIS values before and after anesthesia were almost identical. We noticed a statistically significant difference in the values of the minimum BIS. In patients who received sodium thiopental, this value was lower than the minimum value of BIS in patients who received propofol. Time after which the BIS has reached the minimum value was shorter in patients treated with thiopental (93 s) than in patients who received propofol (140s). The value of the BIS prior to anesthesia (98 v 98) was identical to the value of BIS after anesthesia (98 v 98). Baker et al in their clinical research showed same[17]. Although the BIS value before and after anesthesia were identical, but the BIS value at which managed to make a verbal-logical contact with the sick was lower by 17.6% from baseline (72.4 v 73) in both groups.

Fall asleep time of patients assessed as ciliary reflex decay time didn,t differ significantly in both groups, as well as the time between drug administration and awake. However, BIS recovery time after waking up to pre-sedation value was significantly shorter in patients receiving propofol. This moment was considered the end of the sedation and the patient returned to the clinic of cardiology. Similar acted Baker et al [17]. Time since the recovery of verbal-logical contact with the patient until the return of BIS values to baseline was longer in patients who received sodium thiopental (385 s) than in patients who received propofol. (253 s). Administration of each drug in a single dose was sufficient to realize the ICD tests. Shorter BIS recovery time shows greater utility of propofol than thiopental for use in the sedation to the ICD tests.

12. Conclusions

1. Propofol at a dose of 1.5 mg / kg and thiopental 5 mg / kg provide sufficiently deep sedation for defibrillator testing - cardioverter.
2. Shorter BIS recovery time in patients receiving propofol demonstrates the increased usefulness of this drug for sedation to the ICD tests.
3. Anesthesia for ICD test using thiopental or propofol is safe for patients with low ejection fraction.
4. During sedation with sodium thiopental and propofol, there was no significant hemodynamic differences in patients undergoing ICD tests.
5. BIS is the easiest ability to assess depth of anesthesia because of the ease of implementation and low invasiveness.

13. References

[1] Kleimann RB, Callans DJ, Hook BG, Marchlinski FE "Effectiveness of noninvasive programmed stimulation for initiating ventricular tachyarrhythmias in patients with third-generation implantable cardioverter defibrillators." PACE 1994; 17: 1462-1468

[2] Anderson M, Stein T, Jones S "A simple noninvasive method for induction of ventricular fibrillation in patients with implantable cardiverter defibrillators." Eur Heart J 1993; 14: 167

[3] Sanders WE, Hamrick GL, Herbst MC, Cascio WE, Simpson RJ, Harton JM "Ventricular fibrillation induction using nonsynchronized low energy external shock during rapid ventricular pacing: method of induction when fibrillation mode of ICD fails" PACE 1996; 19: 431-436

[4] Kempa M, Lubiński A, Królak T, Pazdyga A, Zienciuk A, Świątecka G. „Shock on burst - skuteczna, nieinwazyjna metoda indukcji migotania komów u chorych z kardiowerterem-defibrylatorem serca" Folia Cardiol. 2003, 10 (6): 823-827

[5] ACC/AHA/ESC 2006 Guidelines for Management of Patients With Ventricular Arrhythmias and the Prevention of Sudden Cardiac Death: a report of the American College of Cardiology/American Heart Association Task Force and the European Society of Cardiology Committee for Practice Guidelines (writing committee to develop Guidelines for Management of Patients With Ventricular Arrhythmias and the Prevention of Sudden Cardiac Death): developed in collaboration with the European Heart Rhythm Association and the Heart Rhythm Society.Zipes DP, Camm AJ, Borggrefe M, Buxton AE, Chaitman B, Fromer M, Gregoratos G, Klein G, Moss AJ, Myerburg RJ, Priori SG, Quinones MA, Roden DM, Silka MJ, Tracy C, Smith SC Jr, Jacobs AK, Adams CD, Antman EM, Anderson JL, Hunt SA, Halperin JL, Nishimura R, Ornato JP, Page RL, Riegel B, Blanc JJ,

Budaj A, Dean V, Deckers JW, Despres C, Dickstein K, Lekakis J, McGregor K, Metra M, Morais J, Osterspey A, Tamargo JL, Zamorano JL; American College of Cardiology/American Heart Association Task Force; European Society of Cardiology Committee for Practice Guidelines; European Heart Rhythm Association; Heart Rhythm Society. Circulation. 2006 Sep 5;114(10):e385-484. Epub 2006 Aug 25.

[6] ESC guidelines for the diagnosis and treatment of acute and chronic heart failure 2008: the Task Force for the diagnosis and treatment of acute and chronic heart failure 2008 of the European Society of Cardiology. Developed in collaboration with the Heart Failure Association of the ESC (HFA) and endorsed by the European Society of Intensive Care Medicine (ESICM).Dickstein K, Cohen-Solal A, Filippatos G, McMurray JJ, Ponikowski P, Poole-Wilson PA, Strömberg A, van Veldhuisen DJ, Atar D, Hoes AW, Keren A, Mebazaa A, Nieminen M, Priori SG, Swedberg K; ESC Committee for Practice Guidelines (CPG). Eur J Heart Fail. 2008 Oct;10(10):933-89. Epub 2008 Sep 16.

[7] Nawrocka M., Wujtewicz M.A. , Kwiecińska B., Dylczyk-Sommer A., Owczuk R. , Kempa M. : Changes in bispectral index during anaesthesia with a single injection of thiopental or propofol for cardioverter - defibrillator testing: Anaesthesiology Intensive Therapy 2007;39,140-143

[8] Gale DW, Grisson TE, Mirenda JV: Titration of intravenous anesthesia for cardioversion: a com of propofol, metohexital and midazolam. Crit Care Med 1993 : 21(10) :1509 - 13

[9] Sadovsky R.: Deep sedation during cardioversion : American Family Physican : 2004, 70,3

[10] Herregods LL, Bossuyt GP, De Baerdemeaker LE, Moerman AT, Struys MM, Den Blauwen NM, Tavernier RM, Mortier E.: Ambulatory elecrical external cardioversion with propofol or etomidate. J. Clin Anesth, 2003: 15(2) :91-96

[11] Pacifico A., Cedillo - Salazar F. R., Nasir N., Doyle T. K., Henry P. D.: Conscious Sedation with combined hypnotic agents for implantation of implantable cardioverter - defirillators JACC 30(3), 1997: 769 - 73

[12] Lehmann A., Boldt J., Zeitler C., Thaler E., Werling C.: Total intravenous anesthesia with remifentanyl and propofol for implantation of cardioverter - defibrillators in patients with severly reduced left ventricular function . J. Cardiothorac Vasc Anesth. 1999; 13(1):15-9

[13] Tung R.T., Bajaj A.K.: Safety of implantation of cardioverter - defibrillator without general anesthesia in an electrophysiology labolatory. The American Journal of Cardiology 75 (14), 1995, : 908 - 912

[14] Weinbroum A.A., Glick A., Copperman Y., Yashar T., Rudick V., Flaishon R.: Halothane, isoflurane and fentanyl increase the minimally effective defibrillation threshold of an implantable cardioverter defibrillator : first report in Humans . Anesth Analg 2002;95:1147 - 1153

[15] Lipscomb K. J., Linker N. J., Fitzpatrick A. P.: Subpectoral implantation of a cardioverter defibrillator under local anaesthesia, Heart 1998; 79:253-255

[16] Irwin MG, Hui TWC, Milne SE, Kenny GNC: Propofol effective concentrarion 50 and its relationship to bispectral index : Anaesthesia 2002, 57, 242 - 248
[17] Baker GW, Sleigh JW, Smith P: Electroencephalographic indices related to hypnosis and amnesia during propofol anaesthesia for cardioversion: Anaesthesia and Intensive Care: 2000, 28,4